CURRENT CLINICAL STRATEGIES

MEDICINE

Second Edition

Paul D. Chan, M.D.

Michael Safani, Pharm. D.
Assistant Clinical Professor
School of Pharmacy
University of California, San Francisco

Peter J. Winkle, M.D.
University of California, Los Angeles

Nicholas Y. Lorenzo, M.D.
Neurology Editor

Preface

Current Clinical Strategies provides a link between the current medical literature and the hospital wards. For each disease entity covered, the special nursing orders, diagnostic tests, and therapeutic alternatives are presented. It is the most current source for therapeutic strategies available, including up-to-the-minute information on the treatment of AIDS and other modern diseases. This reference provides help for physicians and medical students who would like to write comprehensive admitting orders; it prevents omission of important laboratory tests and therapeutic measures.

This manual is structured to allow the clinician to individualize patient care by selecting diagnostic tests based upon clinical indications, and then to choose the clinically indicated treatment plan from the alternatives provided. Some of the specific orders may not be appropriate for a given patient, and the physician should use his or her own judgement to select orders as required by the clinical picture.

Readers are encouraged to make suggestions by writing to the publisher. Contributors will be acknowledged.

Publishing Information for Authors may be Obtained by Writing to:
Current Clinical Strategies Publishing
9550 Warner Ave, Suite 250
Fountain Valley, California USA 92708-2822
Phone: 800-331-8227; 714-965-9400 Fax: 714-965-9401

Printed in USA   ISBN 1-881528-00-6

CONTENTS

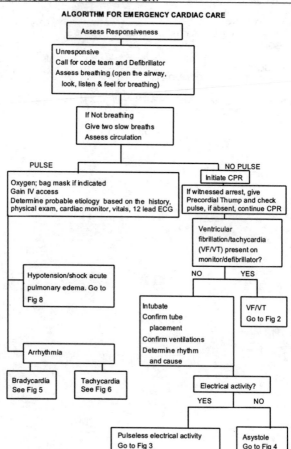

Fig 1 - Algorithm for Adult Emergency Cardiac Care

**ALGORITHM FOR VENTRICULAR FIBRILLATION AND
PULSELESS VENTRICULAR TACHYCARDIA**

Assess Airway, Breathing, Circulation
Perform CPR until defibrillator ready (precordial thump if witnessed arrest)
Ventricular Fibrillation or Tachycardia present on defibrillator

Defibrillate immediately up to 3 times at 200 J, 200-300 J, 360 J.
Do not delay defibrillation

Check pulse and Rhythm

Continue CPR
Gain IV access
Intubate if no response.

| Persistent or recurrent VF/VT | Return of spontaneous circulation | Pulseless Electrical Activity Go to Fig 3 | Asystole Go to Fig 4 |

Continue CPR
Intubate at once
Obtain IV access

Assess vital signs
Support airway
Support breathing

Provide medications appropriate for blood
pressure, heart rate, and rhythm

Epinephrine 1 mg
IV push repeat
q3-5 min or 2 mg in
10 ml NS via ET tube
q3-5 min.
High dose Epinephrine,
0.1 mg/kg IV push,
repeat q3-5 min.
Continue CPR
Defibrillate 360 J

Lidocaine 1.5 mg/kg (100 mg) IV bolus repeat q3-5 min to total
loading dose of 3 mg/kg or dilute in 10 ml NS via ET tube.

CPR for 30-60 sec
Defibrillate 360 J, 30-60 seconds after each dose of medication
Repeat the pattern of drug-shock, drug-shock

Repeat Lidocaine q3-5 min **OR**
Bretylium 10 mg/kg IV bolus q5-10min until max 30 mg/kg.
CPR for 30-60 sec
Defibrillate 360 J

Consider Procainamide 1 gm IV over 30 min, then 1-4 mg/min.
Consider magnesium sulfate 1-2 gm IV if Torsade de Pointes, suspected
hypomagnesemia, or severe refractory VF.
Consider Sodium Bicarbonate 1 mEq/kg IV if long arrest period or hyperkalemia
Repeat pattern of drug-shock, drug-shock

Note: Epinephrine, lidocaine, atropine may be given via endotracheal tube at 2-2.5
times the IV dose. Dilute in 10 cc of saline
After each Intravenous dose, give 20-30 mL bolus of IV fluid & elevate extremity
Fig 2 - Algorithm for Ventricular Fibrillation and Pulseless Ventricular Tachycardia

ALGORITHM FOR PULSELESS ELECTRICAL ACTIVITY

PEA includes   Electromechanical dissociation (EMD)
                Pseudo-EMD
                Idioventricular rhythms
                Ventricular escape rhythms
                Bradyasystolic rhythms
                Postdefibrillation idioventricular rhythms

Initiate CPR, IV access, intubate, assess pulse +/- doppler ultrasound of blood flow

---

Consider possible causes
    Hypoxia (ventilate)
    Hypovolemia (volume infusion)
    Pericardial tamponade (pericardiocentesis)
    Tension pneumothorax (needle decompression)
    Pulmonary embolism (thrombectomy, thrombolytics)
    Drug overdoses (tricyclics, digoxin, beta or calcium
      blockers)
    Hyperkalemia or hypokalemia
    Acidosis (bicarbonate)
    Myocardial infarction (thrombolytics)
    Hypothemia (active rewarming)

Epinephrine 1.0 mg IV bolus q3-5 min or high dose epinephrine
    0.1 mg/kg IV push q3-5 min; may give via ET tube.
Continue CPR

If absolute bradycardia (<60 beats/min) or relative bradycardia,
    give atroprine 1 mg IV, q3-5 min, up to total of 0.04 mg/kg
Consider bicarbonate, 1 mEq/kg IV (1-2 amp, 44 mEq/amp)
    if hyperkalemia or other indications.

Fig 3 - Algorithm for Pulseless Electrical Activity

ALGORITHM FOR ASYSTOLE

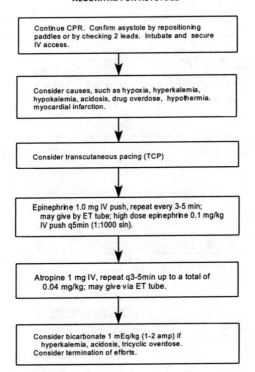

Continue CPR. Confirm asystole by repositioning paddles or by checking 2 leads. Intubate and secure IV access.

Consider causes, such as hypoxia, hyperkalemia, hypokalemia, acidosis, drug overdose, hypothermia. myocardial infarction.

Consider transcutaneous pacing (TCP)

Epinephrine 1.0 mg IV push, repeat every 3-5 min; may give by ET tube; high dose epinephrine 0.1 mg/kg IV push q5min (1:1000 sln).

Atropine 1 mg IV, repeat q3-5min up to a total of 0.04 mg/kg; may give via ET tube.

Consider bicarbonate 1 mEq/kg (1-2 amp) if hyperkalemia, acidosis, tricyclic overdose. Consider termination of efforts.

Fig 4 - Asystole treatment algorithm

ALGORITHM FOR BRADYCARDIA

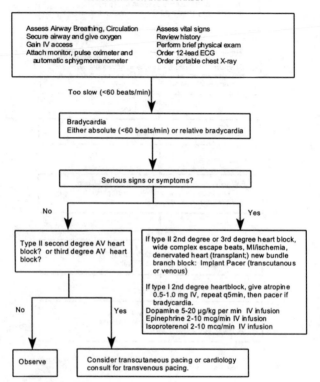

Assess Airway Breathing, Circulation
Secure airway and give oxygen
Gain IV access
Attach monitor, pulse oximeter and
    automatic sphygmomanometer

Assess vital signs
Review history
Perform brief physical exam
Order 12-lead ECG
Order portable chest X-ray

Too slow (<60 beats/min)

Bradycardia
Either absolute (<60 beats/min) or relative bradycardia

Serious signs or symptoms?

No

Yes

Type II second degree AV heart block? or third degree AV heart block?

If type II 2nd degree or 3rd degree heart block, wide complex escape beats, MI/ischemia, denervated heart (transplant;) new bundle branch block: Implant Pacer (transcutaneous or venous)

If type I 2nd degree heartblock, give atropine 0.5-1.0 mg IV, repeat q5min, then pacer if bradycardia.
Dopamine 5-20 µg/kg per min IV infusion
Epinephrine 2-10 mcg/min IV infusion
Isoproterenol 2-10 mcg/min IV infusion

No

Yes

Observe

Consider transcutaneous pacing or cardiology consult for transvenous pacing.

Fig 5 - Bradycardia algorithm (with the patient not in cardiac arrest).

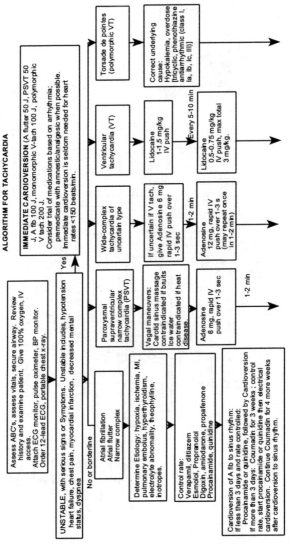

ALGORITHM FOR TACHYCARDIA

Assess ABC's, assess vitals, secure airway. Review history and examine patient. Give 100% oxygen, IV access. Attach ECG monitor, pulse oximeter, BP monitor. Order 12-lead ECG, portable chest x-ray.

UNSTABLE, with serious signs or Symptoms. Unstable includes, hypotension heart failure, chest pain, myocardial infarction, decreased mental status, dyspnea

IMMEDIATE CARDIOVERSION (A. flutter 50 J, A. fib 100 J, PSVT 50 J, A. fib 100 J, monomorphic V-tach 100 J, polymorphic V tach 200 J.
Consider trial of medications based on arrhythmia; premedicate with amnestic/analgesic when possible. Immediate cardioversion is seldom needed for heart rates <150 beats/min.

No or borderline — Yes

Atrial fibrilation / Atrial flutter / Narrow complex

Paroxysmal supraventricular narrow complex tachycardia (PSVT)

Wide-complex tachycardia of uncertain type

Ventricular tachycardia (VT)

Torsade de pointes (polymorphic VT)

Determine Etiology: hypoxia, ischemia, MI, pulmonary embolus, hyperthyroidism, electrolyte abnormality, theophylline, inotropes.

Control rate:
Verapamil, diltiazem
Esmolol, Propranolol
Digoxin, amiodarone, propafenone
Procainamide, quinidine

Vagal maneuvers:
Carotid sinus massage contraindicated if bruits contraindicated if heat disease.

If uncertain if V tach, give Adenosine 6 mg rapid IV push over 1-3 sec

Lidocaine 1-1.5 mg/kg IV push

Correct underlying cause:
Hypokalemia, overdose [tricyclic, phenothiazine antiarrhythmic (class I, Ia, Ib, Ic, III)]

Cardioversion of A fib to sinus rhythm:
If less than 3 days and rate controlled:
Procainamide or quinidine, followed by Cardioversion If more than 3 days: Coumadin for 3 weeks ; control rate, start procainamide or quinidine then electrical cardioversion. Continue Coumadin for 4 more weeks after cardioversion to sinus rhythm.

Adenosine 6 mg, rapid IV push over 1-3 sec

1-2 min

Adenosine 12 mg, rapid IV push over 1-3 s (may repeat once in 1-2 min)

1-2 min

Every 5-10 min

Lidocaine 0.5-0.75 mg/kg IV push, max total 3 mg/kg.

Fig 6

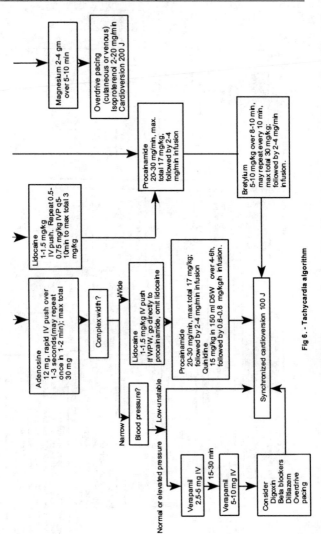

Fig 6. - Tachycardia algorithm

ALGORITHM FOR STABLE TACHYCARDIA

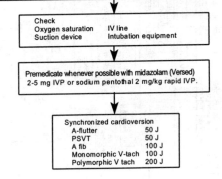

Stable tachycardia with serious signs and symptoms related to the tachycardia. Patient not in cardiac arrest.

If ventricular rate is >150 beats/min, prepare for immediate cardioversion. Immediate cardioversion is generally not needed for rates <150 beats/min. **May give brief trial of medications based on specific arrhythmias.**

V-Tach: Lidocaine 1-1.5 mg/kg IVP, then 0.5-0.75 mg/kg q5-10min to max total 3 mg/kg. If no response, procainamide 20-30 mg/min to max total 17 mg/kg, or Bretylium 5-10 mg/kg over 8-10minutes,q10min to max total 30 mg/kg.

PSVT: Carotid sinus pressure if bruits absent, then adenosine 6 mg rapid IVP, followed by 12 mg rapid IVP x 2 doses to max total 30 mg. If no response, verapamil 2.5-5.0 mg IVP; may repeat dose with 5-10 mg if adequate blood pressure; or Esmolol 500 mcg/kg/min x 1 min, then 50 mcg/kg/min IV infusion, and titrate up to 200 mcg/kg/min IV infusion.

Atrial Fib/Flutter: Digoxin 0.5 mg IVP followed by 0.25 mg IVP q4h x 2-4 doses for rate control, then procainamide 20-30 mg/min IV to total max 17 mg/kg, followed by 2-4 mg/min IV infusion; or quinaglute 15 mg/kg IV over 4-6h, followed by 0.6-0.8 mg/kg/h IV infusion **OR** Diltiazem (rate control only) 0.25 mg/kg IV over 2 min, then 5-15 mg/h IV infusion

Check
Oxygen saturation   IV line
Suction device   Intubation equipment

Premedicate whenever possible with midazolam (Versed) 2-5 mg IVP or sodium pentothal 2 mg/kg rapid IVP.

Synchronized cardioversion
A-flutter   50 J
PSVT   50 J
A fib   100 J
Monomorphic V-tach   100 J
Polymorphic V tach   200 J

Fig 7 - Electrical cardioversion algorithm (with the patient not in cardiac arrest).

ALGORITHM FOR HYPOTENSION, SHOCK, AND ACUTE PULMONARY EDEMA

Patient with clinical signs/symptoms of congestive heart failure, acute pulmonary edema.
Assess ABC's, secure airway, administer oxygen; gain IV access. Monitor ECG, pulse oximeter, BP monitoring.
Check vital signs, review history and examine patient. Order 12-lead ECG, portable chest X-ray.

Determine underlying cause.

Hypovolemia

Administer Fluids, blood
Consider vasopressors, if indicated
Apply hemostasis; treat underlying problem.

Pump Failure

Determine blood pressure

Systolic BP <70 μg/kg

Consider
Norepinephrine 0.5-30 μg/min IV or
Dopamine 5-20 μg/kg per min

Systolic BP 70-100 mm Hg

Dopamine 2.5-20 μg/kg per min IV (add norepinephrine if dopamine is >20 μg/min)

Systolic BP >100 mm Hg and diastolic BP normal

Dobutamine 2.0-20 μg/kg per min IV

Diastolic BP >110 mm Hg

If ischemia and hypertension: nitroglycerin 10-20 μg/min IV, and titrate to effect and/or Nitroprusside 0.1-5.0 μg/kg/min IV

Consider further Therapy

Bradycardia or Tachycardia

Bradycardia Go to Fig 5

Tachycardia Go to Fig 6

First-line actions
Furosemide IV 0.5-1.0 mg/kg
Morphine IV 1-3 mg
Nitroglycerin SL 0.4 mg tab q3-5min x3
Oxygen/intubate as needed

Second-line actions
Nitroglycerin IV (if BP >100 mm Hg): 10-20 mcg/min IV infusion.
Nitroprusside IV (if BP >100 mm Hg): 0.1-5.0 mcg/kg/min IV infusion.
Dopamine (if BP <100 mm Hg): 5-20 mcg/kg/min IV infusion.
Dobutamine (if BP >100 mm Hg): 2-15 mcg/kg/min IV infusion
Milrinone: 50 mcg/kg IV over 10 min, then 0.375-0.75 mcg/kg/min IV infusion
Positive end-expiratory pressure (PEEP)
Continuous positive airway pressure (CPAP)

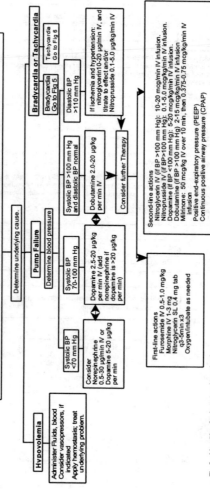

Fig 8 - Algorithm for hypotension, shock, and acute pulmonary edema.

MYOCARDIAL INFARCTION & UNSTABLE ANGINA

1. **Admit to:** Continuously monitored bed (CCU/MICU)
2. **Diagnosis:** Chest pain/rule out MI
3. **Condition:**
4. **Vital signs:** q1h, then q6h. Call MD if pulse >90,<60; BP >150/90, <90/60; R>25, <12; T>38.5°C.
5. **Activity:** Bed rest with bedside commode.
7. **Nursing:** I&O, guaiac stools.
8. **Diet:** Cardiac diet, 1200-1800 cal, 1-2 gm sodium, low fat, low cholesterol diet. No caffeine or temperature extremes.
9. **IV Fluids:** D5W at TKO
10. **Special Medications:**
 -Oxygen 2-4 L/min by NC.
 -Morphine sulfate 2-5 mg slow IV q5-10min until pain free.
 -Nitroglycerine Drip 15 mcg IV bolus, then 10 mcg/min infusion (50 mg in 250-500 ml D5W, 100-200 mcg/ml). Titrate in 5-10 mcg/min steps, up to 200-300 mcg/min; maintain MAP >80 or syst >90; titrate to control symptoms; keep heart rate at less than 20% of baseline rate **OR**
 -Nitroglycerine SL, 0.4 mg (0.15-0.6 mg) SL q5min until pain free (up to 3 tabs)
 -Aspirin 80 or 325 mg PO to chew and swallow, then aspirin E.C. (Ecotrin) 80, 160, 325 mg PO qd.

Beta-Blockers: Contraindicated in presence of CHF.
 -Metoprolol (Lopressor) 5 mg IV q2-5min x 3 doses; then 25 mg PO q6h x 48h, then 100 mg PO q12h, titrate to HR < 60, may give 2 mg IV q2h prn pulse > 70, hold if systolic <90 **OR**
 -Esmolol hydrochloride (Brevibloc) 500 mcg/kg IV over 1 min, then 50 mcg/kg/min IV infusion titrated to HR of <60 (max of 300 mcg/kg/min) **OR**
 -Propranolol 0.1 mg/kg IV divided in 3 doses q5min; followed in 1h by 20-40 mg PO q6-8h (160-240 mg/d), titrate to HR <60 **OR**
 -Atenolol (Tenormin) 5-10 mg IV, then 50-100 mg PO qd, titrate to HR <60 (max 200 mg/d); use caution if heart failure **OR**

Antiarrhythmics:
 -Lidocaine (treatment of ventricular arrhythmias) 75-100 mg (1 mg/kg) IV over 5 min, then 40 mg (0.5 mg/kg) IV over 5 min q8-10min prn until total of 4 mg/kg, then infuse 1.4-3.5 mg/min (20-50 mcg/kg/min; 2 gm in 500 ml of D5W).

Calcium Channel Blockers:
 -Nifedipine (Procardia) 10-40 mg PO/SL tid-qid; max 120 mg/day [10, 20 mg] **OR**
 Procardia XL 30-120 mg PO qd [30, 60, 90 mg].
 -Diltiazem (Cardizem) 30-120 mg PO tid-qid [30,60, 90, 120 mg]; or Diltiazem SR 60-180 mg PO bid [60, 90, 120 mg]; or Diltiazem CD 180-360 mg PO qd [180, 240, 360 mg].
 -Felodipine (Plendil) 5-10 mg PO qd [5,10 mg].
 -Amlodipine (Norvasc) 2.5-10 mg PO qd [2.5, 5, 10 mg].
 -Isradipine (DynaCirc)2.5,-5 mg PO bid [2.5, 5mg].

-Nicardipine (Cardene) 20-40 mg PO tid [20, 30 mg]; or Cardene SR 45-60 mg PO bid [45, 60 mg].

-Bepridil (Vascor) 200-400 mg PO qd [200, 300, 400 mg].

-Verapamil (Calan, Isoptin) 40-120 mg PO q8h [40, 80, 120 mg]; or Verapamil SR 120-240 mg PO qd [120, 180, 240 mg].

Thrombolytic Therapy, see page 17.

Other Medications

-Heparin (if indicated after thrombolysis or PTCA or if CK >700) 5000 U (100 U/kg) IV bolus followed by 1000 U/hr (15 U/kg); adjust to PTT 2-2.5 times control or ACT 200-250 **OR** 5000 units SQ q8-12h.

-Isosorbide dinitrate (Isordil) 10-60 mg PO tid [5,10,20, 30,40 mg]; Sustained release, 40-80 mg PO q8-12h [40 mg] **OR**

-Nitroglycerine ointment (2%) ½-2 inch q4-8h **OR**

-Nitroglycerine Patch (Transderm-Nitro) 0.1-0.6 mg/h qd. If used for more than 24 hours, remove after 8 pm [0.1, 0.2,0.3, 0.4, 0.6 mg/h patches].

-Magnesium Sulfate 4-8 gms in 100-800 cc D5W over 4-8h.

11. Symptomatic Medications:

-Acetaminophen (Tylenol) 325-650 mg PO q4-6h prn headache.

-Lorazepam (Ativan) 1-2 mg PO tid or qid prn anxiety **OR**

-Diphenhydramine (Benadryl) 25-50 mg PO qhs prn sleep.

-Docusate (Colace) 100-250 mg PO bid.

-Dimenhydrinate (Dramamine) 25-50 mg IV over 2-5 min q4-6h or 50 mg PO q4-6h prn nausea **OR**

-Promethazine (Phenergan) 10 mg IV q4h prn nausea.

-Ranitidine (Zantac) 50 mg IV q8h or 150 mg PO bid.

-Mylanta 30 ml PO qid prn heartburn.

12. Extras: ECG stat & in 12h, repeat if chest pain; portable CXR, echocardiogram. Consider cardiology consult for catheterization.

13. Labs: SMA7 & 12, magnesium. Cardiac enzymes: CPK, CPK-MB, STAT & q6h x 24h & qd until peak. LDH & isoenzymes. CBC, fasting LDL, HDL, triglyceride, cholesterol. PT/PTT, lidocaine/drug levels, UA.

14. Other Orders and Meds:

PHARMACOLOGY OF UNSTABLE ANGINA

Drug	Benefits			Disadvantages
	Reduce Mortality	Prevent AMI	Reduce Angina	
Aspirin	+++	+++	---	Bleeding
Heparin	---	+++	++	Bleeding, thrombocytopenia
Nitrates	---	+	+++	Tolerance, hypotension
Beta blockers	---	+	+++	Bronchoconstriction, AV block, reduced contractility
Calcium blockers	---	---	+++	Hypotension, AV block, reduced contractility, tachycardia.
Lytic therapy	---	---	+	bleeding

AMI = acute myocardial infarction; AV = atrioventricular

THROMBOLYTIC THERAPY IN MYOCARDIAL INFARCTION

I. Obtain cardiology consult as soon as possible.

II. **Thrombolytics (chest pain <6 hours)**

Contraindications: Documented bleeding disorder; history of recent GI or GU bleed; BP >200/120; history of recent CVA; head trauma or major surgery (within 2 months); history of prolonged CPR; pregnancy; suspected dissecting aortic aneurysm; hemorrhagic retinopathy.

A. Streptokinase or Anistreplase (APSAC):

1. Aspirin 325 mg chew and swallow now and qd **AND**
   Heparin 5000 U IV push **AND**
   Diphenhydramine 50 mg IV push **AND**
   Methylprednisolone 250 mg IV push.
2. Streptokinase - 1.5 million IU of streptokinase in 100 ml NS IV over 60 min
   OR
   Anistreplase - 30 units IV over 2-5min.
3. Heparin 10 U/kg/h IV immediately after administration of streptokinase or anistreplase and maintain PTT 1.5-2 times control.
4. PTT, fibrinogen now **AND** q6h x 24h. No IM or arterial punctures, watch IV for bleeding.

OR

B. Recombinant tissue plasminogen activator (tPA):

1. Aspirin, 325 mg chew and swallow now & qd. Heparin 5000 U IV bolus
2. Consider beta Blocker Tx.

3. Reconstitute 100 mg tPA (50 mg tPA/vial): tPA 15 mg IVP over 2 min, followed by 0.75 mg/Kg (max 50 mg) IV infusion over 30 min, followed by 0.5 mg/Kg (max 35 mg) IV infusion over 60 min (total dose $\leq$ 100 mg).
4. Start heparin 15 U/kg/h infusion after tPA, & adjust to PTT of 1.5-2 times control.
5. PTT & fibrinogen now & q6h x 24h. No IM or arterial punctures, watch IV for bleeding.

Consider prophylactic IV Lidocaine treatment for reperfusion arrhythmia.

III. Diagnostic Considerations: PT/PTT, thrombin time, FDP, fibrinogen, reptilase time, bleed time, type & screen.

4. Other orders and Meds:

CONGESTIVE HEART FAILURE

1. **Admit to:**
2. **Diagnosis:** Congestive Heart Failure
3. **Condition:**
4. **Vital signs:** q1h. Call MD if P>120; BP >150/100 <80/60; T>38.5°C; R >25 <10.
5. **Activity:** Bed rest with bedside commode.
6. **Nursing:** Daily wts., I&O, Head of bed at 45°, legs elevated.
7. **Diet:** 0.5-2 gm salt cardiac diet. Fluid intake of 1-1.5 L/d.
8. **IV Fluids:** Hep-lock with flush q shift. Foley to closed drainage.
9. **Special Medications:**
   -Oxygen 2-4 L/min by NC.

Diuretics:
   -Furosemide 10-160 mg IV qd or 20-80 mg PO qAM [20,40,80 mg] **OR**
   -Bumetanide (Bumex) 0.5-1 mg IV q2-3h until response; then 0.5-1.0 mg IV q8-24h (max 10 mg/d); or 0.5-2.0 mg PO qAM **OR**
   -Metolazone (Zaroxolyn) 2.5-10 mg PO qd, max 20 mg/d; 30 min before loop diuretic [2.5,5,10 mg].

Digoxin:
   -Digoxin Loading dose (previously undigitalized) 0.25-0.5 mg IV, followed by 0.25 mg IV q6h until a total dose of 0.75-1.0 mg (8-12 mcg/kg lean body weight; 6-10 mcg/kg in renal failure).
   -Digoxin Augmentation (previously digitalized pt) 0.125-0.25 mg IV, may be repeated once after 4h.
   -Digoxin Maintenance - 0.125-0.5 mg PO or IV qd [0.125,0.25, 0.5 mg].

Inotropics:
   -Dopamine 3-15 µg/kg/min IV (400 mg in 250 cc D5W, 1600 µg/ml), titrate to CO >4, CI >2; syst > 90 **AND/OR**
   -Dobutamine 2.5-10 µg/kg/min, max of 14 µg/kg/min (500 mg in 250 ml D5W, 2 µg/ml) **AND/OR**
   -Milrinone (Primacor) 50 mcg/Kg IV over 10 min, followed by 0.375-0.75 (average 0.5) mcg/Kg/min IV infusion (40 mg in 200 mls NS (QS), conc=0.2 mg/ml).

Nitrates and Nitroprusside:
 -Nitroglycerine 10 µg/min IV (50 mg in 250-500 ml D5W); titrated to MAP 70 systolic > 90, max 300 µg/min. (indicated in ↑ pulmonary capillary wedge pressure secondary to acute ischemia) **OR**
 -Isosorbide dinitrate (Isordil) 40 mg PO qid.
 -Nitroprusside sodium 0.1-10 µg/kg/min IV, increase by 0.1-0.2 µg/kg/min; (50 mg in 250-500 ml D5W) titrate to CI >2-4 & CO >4. Indicated in acute LV failure with ↑ SVR ↓ CO ↑ pulmonary capillary wedge pressure. (If used > 3 days, check thiocyanate and cyanide levels.)

ACE Inhibitors:
 -Captopril (Capoten) 6.25-50 mg PO q8h [12.5, 25,50,100 mg] **OR**
 -Enalapril (Vasotec) 1.25-5 mg slow IV push q6h or 2.5-20 mg PO bid [5,10,20 mg] **OR**
 -Lisinopril (Zestril, Prinivil) 5-40 mg PO qd [5,10,20,40 mg].
 -Benazepril (Lotensin) 10-40 mg PO qd, max 80 mg/d [5,10,20,40 mg].
 -Fosinopril (Monopril) 10-40 mg PO qd, max 80 mg/d [10,20 mg].
 -Quinapril (Accupril) Initially 5-10 mg PO qd, then 20-80 mg PO qd in 1 to 2 divided doses [5,10,20,40 mg].
 -Ramipril (Altace) 2.5-10 mg PO qd, max 20 mg/d [1.25,2.5,5,10 mg].

Other Agents and Potassium:
 -Morphine sulfate 5-10 mg IV q2-4h or 1-4 mg IV q5min prn.
 -Levodopa initial dose of 250 mg PO qid, increased as tolerated to 500 mg PO QID **AND** Pyridoxine (vitamin B6) 50 mg PO qd.
 -KCl (Micro-K) 20-60 mEq PO qd.
 -Magnesium Chloride (Slow-Mag) 2-4 tabs/d PO in divided doses [64 mg].

10. Symptomatic Medications:
 -Heparin 5000 U SQ q12h.
 -Docusate sodium 100-200 mg PO qhs.
 -Ranitidine (Zantac) 50 mg IV q8h or 150 mg PO bid.

11. Extras: CXR PA & Lat, ECG now & repeat if chest pain or palpitations, RVG/MUGA, echo, signal averaged ECG.

12. Labs: SMA 7 & 12, CBC, cardiac enzymes, thyroid panel, ABG, iron studies. Repeat SMA 7 & 12 in AM. Digoxin level. UA. Consider thyroid function tests.

13. Other orders and meds:

PAROXYSMAL SUPRAVENTRICULAR TACHYCARDIA

1. Admit to:

2. Diagnosis: PSVT

3. Condition:

4. Vital signs: q1h. Call MD if BP >160/90, <90/60; apical pulse >130, <50; R >25, <10; T>38.5°C

5. Activity: Bedrest with bedside commode.

6. Nursing:

7. Diet: Low fat, low cholesterol, no caffeine.

8. IV Fluids: D5W at TKO.

9. Special Medications:

Attempt vagal maneuvers (Valsalva maneuver and/or carotid sinus massage) before drug therapy (If no bruits).

Cardioversion (if unstable or refractory to drug therapy):

1. NPO x 6h, dig level ≤2.4 & K+ NL.
2. Midazolam (Versed) 2.5 mg IV.
3. If stable, cardiovert with synchronized 10-50 J, increase by 50 J increments. If unstable, start with 75-100 J, then increase to 200 J and 360 J.

Pharmacologic Therapy of PSVT:

-Adenosine (Adenocard) 6 mg rapid IV over 1-2 sec, followed by saline flush, may repeat 12 mg IV after 2-3 min, up to max of 30 mg total (ineffective if on theophylline)

-Verapamil (Isoptin) 2.5-10 mg IV over 2-3min (may give calcium gluconate 1 gm IV over 3-6 min prior to verapamil); then 40-120 mg PO q8h or verapamil SR 120-240 mg PO qd **OR**

-Esmolol hydrochloride (Brevibloc) 500 µg/kg IV over 1 min, then 50 µg/kg/min IV infusion titrated to HR of <60 (max of 300 µg/kg/min) **OR**

-Diltiazem (Cardiazem) 0.25mg/Kg (ave 20 mg) IV over 2 min, then 5-15 mg/hr IV infusion [100 mg/D5W 250 mls (QS); conc 0.4 mg/ml]. For control of ventricular response rate only in atrial fibrillation/flutter.

-Propranolol 1-5 mg (0.15 mg/kg) given IV in 1 mg aliquots min; then 60-80 mg PO tid **OR**

-Digoxin aliquots of 0.25 mg q4h as needed; then 0.125-0.25 mg PO or IV qd **OR**

-Quinidine gluconate (may ↑ AV conduction) 15 mg/kg in 150 ml D5W over 4-6h loading, followed by 0.8 mg/kg/h infusion (reduce dose by 25% if heart failure) **OR** Quinidine sulfate 400 mg PO q 2-4h x 2 doses loading, followed by quinidine gluconate 330 mg IM or PO q8h **OR** quinidine gluconate 330 mg IM or PO q2-4h x 2 doses, then 330 mg IM or PO q8h **OR**

-Procainamide IV loading dose of 1000 mg (15 mg/kg) at 20 mg/min IV; then 2-6 mg/min IV maintenance; or PO loading dose: 750-1000 mg; then 250-1000 mg PO q6h (50 mg/kg/d in 4-6 divided doses) **OR**

-Propafenone (Rythmol) 150-300 mg PO q8h, max 1200 mg/d.

-Flecainide (Tambocor) 50-100 mg PO q12h, max 400 mg/d.

10.Symptomatic Medications:

-Lorazepam (Ativan) 1-2 mg PO tid prn anxiety.

11.Extras: Portable CXR, ECG (rule out Atrial fibrillation/multifocal atrial tachycardia). Repeat if chest pain. Consider cardiology consult for electrophysiologic study if accessory pathway suspected.

12.Labs: CBC, SMA 7 & 12, Mg, UA. ABG, thyroid panel. Drug levels, Quinidine, theophylline, toxicology screen.

13. Other Orders and Meds:

Differential Points Distinguishing Supraventricular Tachycardia (SVT) from Aberrancy from Ventricular Tachycardia (VT)

	VT	SVT w/aberrancy
QRS width	>0.14 sec	<0.14 sec
Axis	Left or bizarre	Normal
V_1	Rs, Rsr', RsR'	rsR'
V_6	S wave present	S wave absent
Fusion beats	Present	Absent
Atrioventricular dissociation	Present	Absent

VENTRICULAR ARRHYTHMIAS

1. **Ventricular Fibrillation & Tachycardia:**
   - **If unstable (see ACLS protocol page 6)**, defibrillate with unsynchronized 200 J, then 300 J.
   - Oxygen 100% by mask.
   - Lidocaine loading dose 75-100 mg IV, then 2-4 mg/min IV **OR**
   - Procainamide loading dose 10-15 mg/kg at 20 mg/min IV or 100 mg IV q5min, then 1-4 mg/min IV maintenance **OR**
   - Bretylium loading dose 5-10 mg/kg over 5-10 min, then 1-4 mg/min IV.
   - **Also see "other antiarrhythmics" below**.

2. **TORSADES DE POINTES:**
   - Correct underlying cause & consider discontinuing quinidine, procainamide, disopyramide, moricizine, lidocaine, amiodarone, phenothiazine & tricyclics, hypokalemia.
   - Magnesium sulfate (drug of choice) 1-4 gm in IV bolus over 5-15 min or infuse 3-20 mg/min for 7-48h until QT interval <0.5 sec.
   - Isoproterenol (Isuprel)(may worsen ischemia) 2-20 µg/min (2 mg in 500 ml D5W, 4 µg/ml) **OR**
   - Phenytoin (Dilantin) 100-300 mg IV given in 50 mg aliquots q5min.
   - Consider ventricular pacing & cardioversion.

3. **Other Antiarrhythmics:**

Class I:
   - Moricizine (Ethmozine) 200-300 mg PO q8h, max 900 mg/d.

Class Ia:
   - Quinidine sulfate 200-600 mg PO q4-6h (max 2.4 gm/d) or gluconate 324-648 mg PO q8-12h **OR**
   - Procainamide PO loading dose of 750-1000 mg (15 mg/kg) in 2-3 divided doses, then 250-1000 mg PO q4-6h or 1 gm IV load given as 100 mg IV q5min or 20 mg/min until arrhythmia suppressed, then 2-6 mg/min IV infusion **OR**
   - Disopyramide 100-300 mg PO q6-8h.

Class Ib:
   - Lidocaine 75-100 mg IV, then 2-4 mg/min IV **OR**
   - Mexiletine (Mexitil) 100-200 mg PO q8h, max 1200 mg/d **OR**

-Tocainide (Tonocard) loading 400-600 mg PO, then 400-600 mg PO q8-12h (1200-1800 mg/d PO in divided doses q8-12h **OR**
-Phenytoin, loading dose 100-300 mg IV given as 50 mg in NS over 10 min IV q5min, then 100 mg IV q5min prn.

Class Ic:
-Flecainide (Tambocor) 50-100 mg PO q12h, max 400 mg/d.
-Propafenone (Rythmol) 150-300 mg PO q8h, max 1200 mg/d.

Class II:
-Propranolol 1-3 mg IV in NS (max 0.15 mg/kg) or 20-80 mg PO q6h (80-160 mg/d) **OR**
-Esmolol loading dose 500 mcg/kg over 1 min, then 50-200 mcg/kg/min IV infusion **OR**
-Atenolol 50-100 mg/d PO **OR**
-Nadolol 40-100 mg PO qd-bid **OR**
-Metoprolol 50-100 mg PO bid-tid **OR**
-Timolol 20 mg/d PO.

Class III:
-Amiodarone (Cordarone) PO loading 400-1200 mg/d in divided doses x 5-14 days, then 200-400 mg PO qd (5-10 mg/kg) **OR**
-Bretylium 5-10 mg/kg IV over 5-10 min, then maintenance of 1-4 mg/min IV or repeat boluses 5-10 mg/kg IV q6-8h; infusion of 1-4 mg/min IV.
-Sotalol (Betapace) 40-80 mg PO bid, max 320 mg/d in 2-3 divided doses.

4. **Extras:** CXR, ECG, echocardiogram, Holter monitor, signal averaged ECG, electrophysiologic study, cardiology consult, ophthalmologic consult (Amiodarone), baseline pulmonary function tests.
5. **Labs:** SMA 7&12, Mg, calcium, CBC, cardiac enzymes, LFT's, ABG, drug levels, thyroid function test, ANA. UA.
6. **Other Orders and Meds:**

_____

HYPERTENSIVE EMERGENCY

1. **Admit to:**
2. **Diagnosis:** Emergency Hypertension
3. **Condition:**
4. **Vital signs:** q30min. Call MD if sudden change in BP >30 mmHg syst; BP syst >200, <90; diast >120, <60; P >120
5. **Activity:** bed rest
6. **Nursing:** Intra-arterial BP monitoring, daily weights, I&O.
7. **Diet:** Clear liquids.
8. **IV Fluids:** D5W at TKO.
9. **Special Medications:**
   -Nitroprusside sodium 0.25-10 µg/kg/min IV (50 mg in 250 ml of D5W), titrate to desired BP. Discontinue if acute fall in BP >30 systolic **OR**
   -Nitroglycerin 5-100 µg/min IV, titrated to desired BP, up to 300 µg/min (50 mg in 250-500 ml D5W) **OR**

-Labetalol (Trandate, Normodyne) 20 mg IV bolus (0.25 mg/kg), then 20-80 mg boluses IV q10-15min titrated to desired BP (max of 300 mg) Infusion of 1.0-2.0 mg/min; then 100-400 mg PO bid **OR**

-Clonidine (Catapres), initial 0.1-0.2 mg PO followed by 0.05-0.1 mg per hour until DBP <115 (Max total dose of 0.8 mg); then 0.1-2.4 mg/d in divided doses bid-tid, max 2.4 mg/d Clonidine patch (Catapres-TTS) 0.1-0.3 mg/24h apply q7 days [0.1,0.2,0.3 mg/24h] **OR**

-Propranolol 1-10 mg load, then 3 mg/h IV, then 80-640 mg/d PO in divided doses **OR**

-Nifedipine (Procardia) 5-20 mg SL or PO (bite & swallow punctured capsule, 0.25-0.5 mg/kg/dose), repeat prn; then 10-30 mg PO q8-6h, max dose of 120 mg/d **OR** extended release (Procardia XL) 30-60 mg PO qd, max 120 mg [30,60,90 mg] **OR**

-Verapamil (Calan) 3-25 mg/h IV infusion, then 40-80 mg PO tid, max 360 mg/d [40,80,120 mg] or Sustained release 120-240 mg PO qd, max 240 mg PO bid [240 mg] **OR**

-Hydralazine (Apresoline) 10-50 mg IV q3-6h (0.1-0.5 mg/kg/dose, max 25 mg), repeat as needed or 10-100 mg PO qid **OR**

-Diazoxide 50-150 mg (1-2 mg/kg) IV over 5-10 sec, repeat q10-15min as needed or 7.5-30 mg/min IV infusion **OR**

-Enalapril (Vasotec) 1.25-5 mg slow IV push q6h, then 2.5-20 mg PO bid **OR**

-Phentolamine (pheochromocytoma), 5-10 mg IV, repeated as needed up to 20 mg. Monoamine oxidase inhibitor with hypertensive crisis 5 mg IV slow push q4-6h (Norepinephrine at bedside to treat hypotension). **OR**

-Trimethaphan camsylate (Arfonad)(dissecting aneurysm) 2-4 mg/min IV infusion (500 mg in 500 ml D5W).

10. Symptomatic Medications:

11. Extras: Portable CXR, ECG, echocardiogram (rule out structural disease of heart, coarctation) renal doppler & scan.

12. Labs: CBC, peripheral smear, SMA 7, calcium, lipid panel, UA with micro. Thyroid panel, 24h urine for vanillylmandelic acid, metanephrine, catecholamines; serum renin, aldosterone. Thiocyanate, Cyanide levels, ESR, ANA, antistreptolysin antibody, urine drug screen.

13. Other Orders and Meds:

SYNCOPE

1. **Admit to:**
2. **Diagnosis:** Syncope
3. **Condition:**
4. **Vital signs:** q1h, postural BP & pulse q12h; Call MD if BP >160/90, <90/60; P >120, <50; R>25, <10
5. **Activity:** Bed rest.
6. **Nursing:** Fingerstick glucose tid, seizure precautions, guaiac stools.
7. **Diet:** Regular
8. **IV Fluids:** D5W at TKO.

9. Special medications:
Vasovagal Syncope:
   -Scopolamine 1.5 mg transdermal patch q3 days.
Postural Syncope:
   -Fludrocortisone 0.1-1 mg/d PO.
10. Extras: portable CXR, ECG, signal averaged ECG, 24h Holter Monitor, exercise stress test, tilt test, EEG, echo cardiogram, carotid duplex scan, CT/MRI, VQ scan.
11. Labs: CBC, SMA 7 & 12, CPK isoenzymes, Mg, Calcium, C-peptide, insulin. Blood alcohol, ABG, serum cortisol, drug levels, thyroid panel. UA, urine drug screen.
12. Other Orders and Meds:

PULMONOLOGY

PULMONARY EMBOLISM

1. **Admit to:**
2. **Diagnosis:** Pulmonary embolism
3. **Condition:**
4. **Vital signs:** q1h x 12h, then qid; Call MD if BP >160/90, <90/60; P >120, <50; R>30, <10; T>38.5°C; O2 sat < 90%
5. **Activity:** Bedrest with bedside commode
6. **Nursing:** Pulse oximeter, guaiac stools, O2 at 2-4L by NC, dipstick urine qd.
7. **Diet:** Regular
8. **IV Fluids:** D5W at TKO.
9. **Special Medications:**

Anticoagulation:
   -Heparin IV bolus 5000-10,000 U (100 U/kg ideal body weight) then 1000-2000 U/h (20 U/kg/h if <70 years, 15 U/kg/h if ≥ 70 [25,000 U in 250 or 500 ml D5W (50-100 U/ml)]; adjust q4-6h to PTT 1.5-2.0 times control (45-75 sec) x 7-10 d. Draw PTT 6 hours after bolus & q4-6h until PTT 1.5-2.5 x control, then qd or q12h. Check PT at initiation of warfarin & qd.
   -Warfarin (Coumadin) 5 -10 mg PO qd x 2-3 d, then 2-5 mg PO qd based on rate of rise of PT. Maintain INR of 2.0-3.0 (INR 3.0-4.5, if recurrent pulmonary embolism). Patients should be adequately heparinized prior to starting coumadin since a mild procoagulant effect may occur during initial days due to depletion of protein C by coumadin.
   -<u>**Anticoagulant overdose**</u> (see page 33)

Streptokinase (symptoms <48h, positive angiogram, & no contraindications. Use only for massive embolism with hemodynamic compromise):
   1. Baseline CBC, PT/PTT, fibrinogen, thrombin time, UA; acetaminophen 650 mg 1-2 tabs PO q4-6h prn; methylprednisolone 250 mg IV, diphenhydramine 50 mg IV.
   2. Streptokinase, 250,000 units IV over 30 min, then 100,000 units/h for 24-72 hours.
   3. Draw PTT, thrombin time, fibrinogen, fibrin split products 4h after start of infusion. If PTT or thrombin time >5 x control, discontinue; if PTT or thrombin time <2 x control, reload with 500,000 units. If PTT <2 x control after 2nd loading dose, discontinue streptokinase, and use heparin or urokinase.
   4. Discontinue infusion after 24h, PTT or thrombin time after 1h. When PTT is <2 times control, initiate <u>**Heparin**</u> infusion at 10 U/kg/h (<u>**no loading dose**</u>) & gradually increase as fibrinogen is restored to maintain PTT 1.5-2.5 x control .

10. **Symptomatic Medications:**
   -Meperidine 25-100 mg IV prn pain <u>**OR**</u>
   -Morphine Sulfate infusion 0.03-0.05 mg/kg/h continuous IV infusion (50-100 mg in 500 ml D5W) titrated to pain.
   -Docusate sodium (Colace) 100-200 mg PO qhs.
   -Ranitidine (Zantac) 150 mg PO bid.

11. Extras: CXR PA & LAT, ECG, VQ scan, impedance plethysmography, doppler scan of legs, venography, pulmonary angiography, digital subtraction angiography.

12. Labs: CBC, PT/PTT, SMA7, ABG, cardiac enzymes. UA with micro. PTT 6 hours after bolus & q4-6h until PTT 1.5-2.5 x control, then qd or q12h. PT at initiation of warfarin & qd. Consider beta HCG, lupus anticoagulant, protein C anticardiolipin.

13. Other Orders and Meds:

ASTHMA

1. Admit to:

2. Diagnosis: Exacerbation of asthma/status asthmaticus

3. Condition:

4. Vital signs: q1h; measure pulsus paradoxus. Call MD if P >140; R>30, <10; T>38.5°C; O2 Sat < 90%

5. Activity:

6. Nursing: Peak flow rate pre & post bronchodilator treatments, pulse oximeter.

7. Diet: Regular, no caffeine.

8. IV Fluids: D5½NS, at 125 cc/h.

9. Special Medications:
-Oxygen 2-6 L/min by NC. Keep O2 sat >90%.

Beta Agonists, Acute Treatment:
-Albuterol (Ventolin) or Metaproterenol nebulized, 0.2-0.5 ml (2.5 mg) in 3 ml saline initially, then q2-8h (5 mg/ml sln) **OR**
-Albuterol (Ventolin) or Metaproterenol (Alupent) MDI 3-8 puffs, then 1 puffs q1-10min initially. Then 2 puffs q1-6h or powder 200 mcg/capsule inhaled qid. Beta agonists should be changed to prn when patient has stabilized.

Aminophylline & Theophylline:
-Aminophylline load dose: 5.6 mg/kg **total** body weight in 100 ml D5W IV over 20min. Maintenance of 0.5-0.6 mg/kg **ideal** body weight/h (500 mg in 250 ml D5W); reduce if elderly, heart/liver failure (0.2-0.4 mg/kg/hr); may need up to 0.8-0.9 mg/kg/h if smoker. Reduce load 50-75% if taking theophylline (1 mg/kg of aminophylline will raise levels 2 μg/ml) **OR**
-Theophylline IV solution loading dose 4.5 mg/kg **total** body weight, then 0.4-0.5 mg/kg **ideal** body weight/hr.
-Theophylline (Theo-Dur) PO loading dose of 6 mg/kg, then maintenance of 100-400 mg PO bid-tid (3 mg/kg q8h); 80% of total daily IV aminophylline in 2-3 doses.

Corticosteroids:
-Methylprednisolone (Solu-Medrol) 60-125 mg IV q6h; then 30-60 mg PO qd. **OR**
-Prednisone 20-60 mg PO qAM.
-Beclomethasone (Beclovent)(when off IV steroids) MDI 2-6 puffs qid, with spacer 5min after bronchodilator, followed by gargling with water **OR**

-Triamcinolone (Azmacort) MDI 1-4 puffs tid-qid **OR**
-Flunisolide (Aerobid) MDI 2-4 puffs bid.
-Budesonide 200-800 µg qid MDI (50 µg/puff or 250 µg/puff).
-After stabilization, inhaled corticosteroids should be the mainstay of treatment.

Magnesium & Adjunct Pharmacologic Support:
-Pirbuterol (Maxair) MDI 2 puffs q4-6h **OR**
-Bitolterol (Tornalate) MDI 2-3 puffs q1-3min initially, then 2-3 puffs q4-8h **OR**
-Fenoterol (Berotec) MDI 3 puffs initially, then 2 bid-qid.
-Isoetharine (Bronkosol) 0.25-0.5 ml of 1% sln in 2 ml normal saline nebulized q4h. MDI 2 puffs q 3-4h.
-Albuterol 2-4 mg PO tid-qid or albuterol repetab 4-8 mg PO bid (max 24 mg/d).
-Ketotifen (Zaditen) 1-2 mg PO bid or slow release formula, 2 mg PO qd.
-Magnesium sulfate 2 gms in D5W 50 mls over 20 min, if inadequate response to bronchodilators and steroids.

Children & Young Adults:
-Epinephrine (1:1000 sln) 0.01 ml/kg/dose SQ, (max 0.2 mg) q20min x 1-2 doses **OR**
-Terbutaline 0.25 ml (0.25 mg) SQ q3-4h.

Acute Bronchitis
-Ampicillin/sulbactam (Unasyn) 1.5 gm IV q6h **OR**
-Ampicillin 0.5-1 gm IV q6h or 250-500 mg PO qid **OR**
-Bactrim DS, 1 tab PO bid x 7-10 days **OR**
-Amoxicillin/clavulanate (Augmentin) 250-500 mg PO q8h **OR**
-Cefaclor (Ceclor) 250-500 mg PO q8h.

11. Symptomatic Medications:
-Docusate sodium (Colace) 100-200 mg PO qhs.
-Ranitidine (Zantac) 50 mg IV q8h or 150 mg PO bid.

12. Extras: Portable CXR, pulmonary function test with bronchodilators, ECG, skin allergy testing, PPD, pulmonary rehabilitation.

13. Labs: ABG, CBC, SMA7. Phosphorous, Theo level stat & after 24h of infusion & after 24-48h of PO (repeat theo level after 5-6 half lives for long-acting preparations). Serum precipitins IgG to aspergillus fumigatus. Sputum Gram stain, C&S. Eosinophile count. IgE levels, RAST.

14. Other Orders and Meds:

CHRONIC OBSTRUCTIVE PULMONARY DISEASE

1. Admit to:
2. Diagnosis: Exacerbation of COPD
3. Condition:
4. Vital signs: q4h. Call MD if P >130; R>30, <10; T>38.5°C; O2 Sat < 90%.
5. Activity: Bed rest, up in chair if able, bedside commode.
6. Nursing: Peak flow rate pre & post bronchodilators, pulse oximeter.
7. Diet: Regular, no caffeine.

8. IV Fluids: D5½NS with 20 mEq KCL/L at 125 cc/h.

9. Special Medications:
-O2 1-2 L/min by NC or 24-35% by Venturi mask, keep O2 saturation 90-91%.

Beta Agonists, Acute Treatment:
-Nebulized Albuterol (Ventolin) or Metaproterenol (Alupent) 0.2-0.5 ml in 3 ml (2.5 mg) of saline q20min initially, then q2-8h (5 mg/ml sln) **OR**
-Albuterol (Ventolin) or Metaproterenol (Alupent) MDI 2-8 puffs then 2 puffs q10-20 min, with spacer; then 2 puffs q4-6h **OR**
-Isoetharine (Bronkosol) 0.25-0.5 ml of 1% sln in 2 ml NS nebulized q4h. MDI 2 puffs q3-4h. Taper beta agonists to prn when patient has stabilized.

Aminophylline & Theophylline:
-Aminophylline loading dose - 5.6 mg/kg **total** body weight over 20 min (if not already on theophylline preparations); then 0.5-0.6 mg/kg **ideal** body weight/hr (500 mg in 250 ml of D5W at 20 cc/h); reduce if elderly, or heart or liver disease (0.2-0.4 mg/kg/hr). Reduce loading to 50-75% if already taking theophylline (1 mg/kg of aminophylline will raise levels by 2 µg/ml) **OR**
-Theophylline IV solution loading dose 4.5 mg/kg **total** body weight, then 0.4-0.5 mg/kg **ideal** body weight/hr.
-Theophylline long acting (Theo-Dur) PO loading dose of 6 mg/kg, then maintenance of 100-400 mg PO bid-tid (3 mg/kg q8h); 80% of daily IV aminophylline in 2-3 doses.

Corticosteroids & Anticholinergics:
-Methylprednisolone (Solu-Medrol) 40-60 mg IV q6h or 30-60 mg PO qd **Followed by:**
-Prednisone 20-40 mg PO qd, taper to minimum dose (taper to 5-10 mg per week).
-Triamcinolone (Azmacort) MDI 2-4 puffs qid **OR**
-Beclomethasone (Beclovent) MDI 2-6 puffs qid, with spacer, 5 min after bronchodilator, followed by gargling with water **OR**
-Flunisolide (Aerobid) MDI 2-4 puffs bid.
-Atropine 1-2 mg in 1 cc NS by nebulizer q4h **OR**
-Ipratropium Bromide (Atrovent) MDI 2 puffs tid-qid.

Acute Bronchitis
-Ampicillin 1 gm IV q6h or 250-500 mg PO qid **OR**
-Trimethoprim/Sulfamethoxazole (Septra DS) 160/800 mg PO bid or 160/800 mg DS IV q8-12h (6-10 mg TMP/kg/d)(10-15 ml of IV sln in 100 cc D5W tid; 16 mg/ml) **OR**
-Ampicillin/sulbactam (Unasyn) 1.5 gm IV q6h **OR**
-Cefuroxime 1.5 gm IV q8h **OR**

10. Symptomatic Medications:
-Docusate sodium (Colace) 100-200 mg PO qhs.
-Ranitidine (Zantac) 50 mg IV q8h or 150 mg PO bid.

11. Extras: Portable CXR, PFT's with bronchodilators, ECG, PPD with controls.

12. Labs: ABG, CBC, phosphorus, SMA7. UA. Theo level stat & after 12-24h of infusion & 24h after PO. Sputum Gram stain & C&S.; alpha 1 antitrypsin level

13. Other Orders and Meds:

HEMOPTYSIS

1. **Admit to:**
2. **Diagnosis:** Hemoptysis
3. **Condition:**
4. **Vital signs:** q1h; Orthostatic BP & pulse bid. Call MD if BP >160/90, <90/60; P >130, <50; R>25, <10; T>38.5°C; O2 sat <90%
5. **Activity:** Bed rest with bedside commode. Keep patient lateral decubitus Trendelenburg, bleeding side down.
6. **Nursing:** Quantify all sputum & blood, suction prn. Endotracheal tube (8 mm) ready, O2 at 100% by mask, pulse oximeter. Discontinue narcotics & sedatives.
7. **Diet:**
8. **IV Fluids:** NS at 0.5-1 L/hr x 1-3 L (≥16 gauge), then transfuse PRBC, Foley to gravity.
9. **Special Medications:**
   -Transfuse 2-6 U PRBC over 2-6h.
   -Codeine (cough suppression may be contraindicated if massive hemoptysis) 15-30 mg PO q4-6h **OR**
   -Hydrocodone 5 mg PO q4-6h.
10. **Other Considerations:**
    -Have double lumen endotracheal tube available for use; consult an anesthesiologist or pulmonologist experienced in double lumen tube placement if necessary. Consider empiric antibiotics if any suggestion that bronchitis or infection may be contributing to hemoptysis.
11. **Extras:** CXR PA, LAT & lordotic, ECG, VQ scan, contrast CT, technetium scan, bronchoscopy. PPD & controls, pulmonary & thoracic surgery consults.
12. **Labs:** type & cross 4-6 U PRBC. ABG, CBC, platelets, SMA7 & 12, ESR, Anti-glomerular basement antibody, rheumatoid factor, immunoglobulins, complement, cryoglobulins, anti-nuclear cytoplasmic antibody. Sputum Gram stain, C&S, AFB, parasites & fungal, & cytology x 3, sputum pH. UA, PT/PTT, von Willebrand Factor, factor 8. Repeat CBC q6h x 24h.
13. **Other Orders and Meds:**

ANAPHYLAXIS

1. **Admit to:**
2. **Diagnosis:** Anaphylaxis
3. **Condition:**
4. **Vital signs:** q1h; Call MD if BP syst >160, <90; diast. >90, <60; P >120, <50; R>25, <10; T>38.5°C
5. **Activity:** Bedrest
6. **Nursing:** I&O q1h, O2 at 6 L/min by NC or mask. Place patient in Trendelenburg's position, No. 4 or 5 endotracheal tube at bedside, FEV 1, peak flow q20min.
7. **Diet:** NPO
8. **IV Fluids:** 2 IV lines. Normal saline or LR 1-6 L over 1-2 h, then D5½NS at 150-200 cc/h. Foley to closed drainage.
9. **Special Medications:**

Gastrointestinal Decontamination:
   -Gastric lavage if indicated.
   -Activated charcoal 50-100 gm, followed by cathartic.

Bronchodilators:
   -Epinephrine (1:1000) 0.3-0.5 ml SQ or IM q10min or 1-4 mcg/min IV **OR** in severe life threatening reactions give 0.5 mg (5.0 mL of 1: 10,000 sln) IV q5-10min prn. **OR** dilute in 10 mL NS & give via endotracheal tube; Epinephrine, 0.3 mg of 1:1000 sln may be injected SQ at site of allergen injection) **OR**
   -Aerosolized 2% racemic Epinephrine 0.5-0.75 ml **OR**
   -Terbutaline, 1 mg (1 ml) in 2 cc NS by nebulizer.
   -Albuterol (Ventolin) 0.5%, 0.5 mL in 2.5 mL NS q20min by nebulizer.
   -Aminophylline loading dose 5.6 mg/kg **total** body weight IV, then infuse 0.3-0.9 mg/kg **ideal** body weight/h **OR**
   -Theophylline IV solution, loading dose 4.5 mg/kg **total** body weight, then 0.4-0.5 mg/kg **ideal** body weight/hr.
   -Atropine sulfate 1 mg in 2.5 mL of NS q4h by nebulizer or 0.8-1 mg IV q2-3 min if bradycardia persists (max 3 mg).

Antihistamines:
   -Diphenhydramine (Benadryl) 25-50 mg IV, IM or PO q2-4h **OR**
   -Hydroxyzine 25-50 mg IV, IM or PO q2-4h.
   -Cimetidine (Tagamet) 300 mg IV, IM or PO q6h. **OR**
   -Ranitidine (Zantac) 150 mg IV q12h

Corticosteroids:
   -Methylprednisolone (Solu-Medrol) 50 mg IV q4-6h. **OR**
   -Hydrocortisone Sodium Succinate 200-500 mg IV q4-6h or 70-120 mg/h (300-500 mg in 250 ml D5W at 60 ml/h)(IV steroids should be followed by PO steroids).
   -Prednisone PO 60 mg PO q6h.

Pressors & other Agents:
  -Norepinephrine (Levophed) 8-12 mcg/min IV, adjust to systolic 100 mmHg (8 mg in 500 ml D5W) **OR**
  -Isoproterenol (Isuprel) 0.5-5 mcg/min IV **OR**
  -Dopamine (Intropin) 5-20 µg/kg/min IV.
  -Albumin 25 gm IV (100 mL of 25% sln) **OR**
  -Hetastarch (Hespan) 500-1,000 cc over 30-60 min (max 20 ml/kg or 1500 ml/d).
  -Glucagon 10 mg IV bolus, then infuse 2-8 mg/h IV.

Premedication for radiocontrast or blood products in allergic patient
  -Prednisone 50 mg PO q6h x 3 doses **AND**
  -Diphenhydramine 50 mg IV or PO 1h before procedure.

10. Extras: portable CXR, lateral soft tissue neck x-rays, ECG, pulmonary function test.

11. Labs: CBC, SMA 7&12, ABG, skin testing, radioallergosorbent test (RAST), serum tryptase, complement, C1 inhibitor; urine/plasma histamine, 24h urine for 5-hydroxyindoleacetic acid (carcinoid), UA.

12. Other Orders and Meds:

PLEURAL EFFUSION

1. Admit to:

2. Diagnosis: Pleural effusion

3. Condition:

4. Vital signs: q shift; Call MD if BP >160/90, <90/60; P>120, <50; R>25, <10; T>38.5°C

5. Activity:

6. Diet: 2-3 gm salt diet.

7. IV Fluids: D5W at TKO

8. Nursing: Oxygen 2-6 L/min by NC or mask

9. Extras: CXR PA & LAT repeat after thoracentesis; bilateral lateral decubitus, ECG, ultrasound; PPD & candida, mumps; pulmonary consult.

10. Labs: CBC, ABG, SMA 7 & 12, protein, albumin, amylase, rheumatoid factor, ANA, ESR, PT/PTT, UA. Fungal serologies.

Pleural fluid:
  Tube 1 - LDH, protein, amylase, triglyceride, glucose (10 ml). If turbid then send: cholesterol crystals (rule out chyliform effusion); chylomicrons (rule out chylothorax).
  Tube 2 - Gram stain, C&S, AFB, fungal C&S, wet mount (20-60 ml, heparinized), pH.
  Tube 3 - Cell count and differential (5-10 ml, EDTA).

Tube 4 - Sudan stain, LE prep, antigen tests for S pneumoniae, H influenza, rheumatoid factor, ANA, complement C3, hyaluronic acid (25-50 ml, heparinized).

Syringe - pH (2 ml collected anaerobically, heparinized on ice)

Bag or Bottle - cytology.

10. Other Orders and Meds:

HEMATOLOGY

ANTICOAGULANT OVERDOSE

Heparin Overdose:
1. Discontinue Heparin infusion
2. Protamine sulfate, 1 mg IV for every 100 units of heparin infused in preceding 2h, dilute in 25-50 ml fluid IV over 10-20 min (max 50 mg in 10 min period). Watch for signs of anaphylaxis, especially if patient has been on NPH insulin therapy.

Warfarin (Coumadin) Overdose:
-Gastric lavage & activated charcoal if recent oral ingestion. Discontinue Coumadin and heparin; follow HCT q 1h.

Minor bleeds:
-Vitamin K (Phytonadione), 5-10 mg PO or 2.5-5 mg SQ or 10 mg IV doses titrated to desired PT (q12h until stable).

Serious bleeds:
-Vitamin K (Phytonadione), 10-20 mg in 50-100 ml fluid IV over 30-60 min (PT q6h until stable) **OR**
-Fresh frozen plasma, 2-3 units (severe bleeds).

Labs: CBC, check platelets (if <50,000, transfuse 4-6 U platelets).
Other orders and meds:

DEEP VEIN THROMBOSIS

1. **Admit to:**
2. **Diagnosis:** Deep vein thrombosis
3. **Condition:**
4. **Vital signs:** q shift; Call MD if BP syst >160, <90 diast. >90, <60; P >120, <50; R>25, <10; T>38.5°C.
5. **Activity:** Bed rest with legs elevate.
6. **Nursing:** Guaiac stools, warm packs to leg prn, dipstick urine for blood, measure calf circumference qd, no IM injections or aspirin products.
7. **Diet:** Regular
8. **IV Fluids:** D5W at TKO
9. **Special Medications:**

Anticoagulation:
-Heparin IV bolus 5000-10,000 U (100 U/kg ideal body weight) then 1000-2000 U/h (20 U/kg/h if <70 years, 15 U/kg/h if ≥ 70 [25,000 U in 250 or 500 ml D5W (50-100 U/ml)]; adjust q6h to PTT 1.5-2 times control (50-70 sec) x 5-7 d (baseline labs, see below).
-Warfarin (Coumadin) 5-10 mg PO qd x 2-3 d, then titrate based on rate of rise of PT; maintain INR 2.0-3.0 (INR 3.0-4.5 if recurrent thromboses). May initiate Coumadin on second day of heparin as long as PTT prolonged; discontinue heparin when PT is therapeutic.

10. Symptomatic Medications:
-Propoxyphene/acetaminophen (Darvocet N100) 1-2 tab PO q3-4h prn pain.
-Docusate sodium (Colace) 100-200 mg PO qhs.
-Ranitidine (Zantac) 150 mg PO bid.

5. Extras: CXR PA & LAT, ECG, impedance plethysmography & doppler scan of legs, radiolabeled fibrinogen scan, B-mode ultrasound, duplex scan, venography. V/Q scan.

6. Labs: CBC & PT/PTT, SMA 7. UA with micro. PTT 6h after bolus & q4-6h until PTT 1.5-2.0 x control then qd or q12h. PT at initiation of warfarin & qd. Beta HCG. If recurrent thrombosis or refractory thrombosis on adequate anticoagulation then check: antithrombin III; protein CIE; lupus anticoagulant; anticardiolipin.

7. Other Orders and Meds:

SICKLE CELL CRISIS

1. Admit to:

2. Diagnosis: Sickle Cell Crisis

3. Condition:

4. Vital signs: q shift; call MD if:

5. Activity: Bedrest

6. Nursing:

7. Diet: NPO, advance to clear liquids as tolerated.

8. IV Fluids: D5½NS at 1.5-2.0 x maintenance or 150-250 ml/h.

9. Special Medications:
-Oxygen 2-4 L/min by NC or 30-100% by mask; consider hyperbaric oxygen therapy; investigational.
-Meperidine (Demerol) 50-150 mg IM/IV/SC q3-4h.
-Hydroxyzine (Vistaril) 25-100 mg IM/IV/PO q3-4h prn pain.
-Morphine sulfate 10 mg IV/IM/SC q2-4h prn **OR** follow bolus by infusion of 0.05-0.1 mg/kg/h or 10-30 mg PO q4h **OR**
-Codeine 15-60 mg IM/SC/PO q4-6h **OR**
-Oxycodone (Roxicodone) 5 mg PO q6h prn **OR**
-Hydromorphone 1-4 mg IM/SC/IV q4-6h or 2-4 mg PO q4-6h prn.
-Acetaminophen/codeine (Tylenol 3) 1-2 tabs PO q4-6h prn.
-Folic acid 1 mg PO qd.
-Transfusion (if indicated)
-Penicillin V (prophylaxis), 250 mg PO bid [tabs 125,250,500 mg].

Vaccination (especially if splenectomized):
-Pneumovax (23V) before discharge 0.5 cc IM x 1 dose; once in a lifetime.
-Influenza vacc (Fluogen) 0.5 cc IM once a year.

10. Extras: CXR, technetium spleen scan, indium scan.

11. Labs: CBC, blood C&S, reticulocyte count, type & hold, direct & indirect bilirubin, sickle prep, Hb electrophoresis, parvovirus titers, SMA 7, UA, urine C&S.

12. Other Orders and Meds:

INFECTIOUS DISEASES

EMPIRIC THERAPY OF MENINGITIS

1. **Admit to:**
2. **Diagnosis:** Meningitis / encephalitis
3. **Condition:**
4. **Vital signs:** q1h; Call MD if BP syst >160/90, <90/60; P >120, <50; R>25, <10; T>39°C or less than 36°C
5. **Activity:** Bed rest with bedside commode.
6. **Nursing:** Respiratory isolation. I&O, daily weights, lumbar puncture tray at bedside. Keep room dark, if viral meningitis with photo sensitivity.
7. **Diet:**
8. **IV Fluids:** D5W at TKO
9. **Special Medications:** (IV Tx x 10-14 d except in Listeria)

Meningitis Empiric Therapy 15-50 years old

  -Penicillin G 3-4 million Units IV q4h (with 3rd gen cephalosporin) **OR**
  -Ampicillin 2 gm IV q4h (with 3rd gen cephalosporin) **AND EITHER**
    Ceftriaxone (Rocephin) 2 gm IV q12h (max 4 gm/d) **OR**
    Cefotaxime (Claforan) 2 gm IV q4h **OR**
    Ceftizoxime (Cefizox) 2 gm IV q4h **OR**
    Ceftazidime (Fortaz) 2 gm IV q4h
  -Consider dexamethasone IV.

Empiric Therapy >50 years old, Alcoholic, Corticosteroids or Hematologic malignancy or other Debilitating Condition:

  -Ampicillin 2 gm IV q4h or penicillin G **AND EITHER**
    Cefotaxime (Claforan) 2 gm IV q4h **OR**
    Ceftriaxone (Rocephin) 2 gm IV q12h (max 4 g/d) **OR**
    Ceftizoxime (Cefizox) 2 gm IV q4h **OR**
    Ceftazidime (Fortaz) 2 gm IV q4h
  -Consider dexamethasone IV.

10. **Symptomatic Meds:**
  -Acetaminophen 325-650 mg PO/PR q4-6h prn temp >101.
11. **Extras:** CXR, ECG, PPD with controls; CT/MRI scan of head.
12. **Labs:** CBC, SMA 7 & 12, osmolality. Blood C&S x 2. UA with micro, urine C&S. Stool, throat, nasal C&S. Antibiotic levels peak & trough after 3rd dose.

  CSF Tube 1 - Glucose, protein (1-2 ml).
  CSF Tube 2 - Gram stain of fluid or sediment (if fluid is clear), C&S for bacteria (1-4 ml).
  CSF Tube 3 - Cell count & differential (1-2 ml).
  CSF Tube 4 - Latex agglutination or counterimmunoelectrophoresis antigen tests for S. pneumoniae, H. influenzae (type B), N. meningitides, E. coli, group B strep, cryptococcus, viral cultures, VDRL (8-10 ml).

13. **Other Orders and Meds:**

INFECTIVE ENDOCARDITIS

1. **Admit to:**
2. **Diagnosis:** Infective endocarditis
3. **Condition:**
4. **Vital signs:** q4h; Call MD if BP syst >160/90, <90/60; P >120, <50; R>25, <10; T>38.5°C
5. **Activity:** Up ad lib
6. **Diet:** Regular
7. **IV Fluids:** Hep-lock with flush q shift.
8. **Special Medications:**

Subacute Bacterial Endocarditis Empiric Therapy:
-Penicillin G 2-3 million U IV q4h or ampicillin 2 gm IV q4h **AND**
Gentamicin 80 mg (1-1.5/mg/kg) IV q8h

Acute Bacterial Endocarditis Empiric Therapy
(including IV drug abuser):
-Gentamicin 100-120 mg IV (2 mg/kg); then 80 mg (1-1.5 mg/kg) IV q8h **AND EITHER**
Nafcillin or Oxacillin 2 gm IV q4h **OR**
Vancomycin 500 mg IV q6h or 1 gm IV q12h (1 gm in 250 ml D5W over 1h q12h).

Streptococci viridans/bovis:
-Penicillin G 2-3 million U IV q4h for 4 weeks **OR**
-Vancomycin 1 gm IV q12h x 4 weeks **AND**
Gentamicin 70 mg (1 mg/kg) q8h for first 2 weeks.

Enterococcus:
-Gentamicin 70 mg (1 mg/kg) IV q8h x 4-6 weeks **AND EITHER**
Penicillin G 3-5 million U IV q4h x 4-6 weeks **OR**
Ampicillin 2 gm IV q4h x 4-6 weeks.

Staphylococcus aureus (methicillin sensitive, native valve):
-Nafcillin or Oxacillin 2 gm IV q4h x 4-6 weeks **OR**
Vancomycin 1 gm IV q12h x 4-6 weeks **AND**
Gentamicin 70 mg (1 mg/kg) IV q8h for first 3-5 days.

Methicillin resistant Staphylococcus aureus (native valve):
-Vancomycin 500 mg IV q6h or 1 gm IV q12h (1 gm in 250 ml D5W over 1h q12h) x 4-6 weeks.

Staphylococcus epidermidis (native valve):
-Vancomycin 500 mg IV q6h or 1 gm q12h x 4-6 weeks **AND**
Gentamicin 70 mg (1 mg/kg) q8h for first 3-5 days **AND**
Rifampin 600 mg PO qd x 6 weeks.

Methicillin sensitive Staph aureus (prosthetic valve):
-Nafcillin or oxacillin 2 gm IV q4h x 6 weeks **AND**
Rifampin 600 mg PO qd x 6 weeks **AND**
Gentamicin 1 mg/kg IV q8h x 2 weeks.

Methicillin resistant Staph aureus (prosthetic valve):
-Vancomycin 500 mg IV q6h or 1 gm IV q12h x 6 weeks **AND**
Rifampin 600 mg PO qd x 6 weeks **AND**
Gentamicin 1 mg/kg IV q8h x 2 weeks.

Staph epidermidis (prosthetic valve):
-Vancomycin 500 mg IV q6h or 1 gm IV q12h x 6 weeks **AND**
Rifampin 600 mg PO qd x 6 weeks **AND**
Gentamicin 1 mg/kg IV q8h x 2 weeks.

Culture Negative Endocarditis:
-Penicillin G 2-3 million U IV q4h x 4-6 weeks **OR**
-Ampicillin 2 gm IV q4h x 4-6 weeks **AND**
Gentamicin 80 mg (1-1.5 mg/kg) q8h x 2 weeks (or use nafcillin and gentamicin if Staph aureus suspected in drug abuser or prosthetic valve).

Fungal Endocarditis:
-Amphotericin B 0.5 mg/kg/d IV (after test dose) + flucytosine 150 mg/kg/d PO.

9. Extras: CXR PA & LAT, M-mode & 2-dimensional echo, ECG, abdominal ultrasound, ECG & repeat q week.

11. Labs: CBC with diff, SMA 7 & 12, liver panel, ESR. Blood C&S x 3-4 over 24h (if septic, draw over 1h) (before starting antibiotic), serum cidal titers, minimum inhibitory concentration, minimum bactericidal concentration. Gram stain C&S of sputum. Repeat C&S in 48h, then q week. Antibiotic levels peak & trough at 3rd dose. UA, urine C&S.

12. Other Orders and Meds:

EMPIRIC THERAPY OF PNEUMONIA

1. **Admit to:**
2. **Diagnosis:** Pneumonia
3. **Condition:**
4. **Vital signs:** q4h; Call MD if BP >160/90, <90/60; P>120, <50; R>25, <10; T>38.5°C or O2 saturation <90%.
5. **Activity:**
6. **Nursing:** Pulse oximeter, I&O, Nasotracheal suctioning prn, incentive spirometry.
7. **Diet:** Regular, push fluids (unless aspiration pneumonia).
8. **IV Fluids:** IV D5½NS at 125 cc/hr or TKO.
9. **Special Medications:**
   -Oxygen by NC at 2-4 L/min or 24-50% Ventimask or 100% non-rebreather (reservoir).

Community Acquired Pneumonia 5-40 years old without underlying lung disease:
-Clarithromycin (Biaxin) 250-500 mg PO bid 7-10 days **OR**
-Azithromycin (Zithromax) 500 mg PO x 1, then 250 mg PO qd x 4 days (T½ 60 hours). **OR**
-Erythromycin (Eramycin) 500 mg IV qid **OR**
-Cefuroxime 25 mg/kg IV q8h (children) or 0.75-1.5 gm IV q8h (adults) **OR**
-Ampicillin/sulbactam (Unasyn) 1.5-3.0 gm IV q6h.

Community Acquired Pneumonia >40 years old:
-Erythromycin 500 mg IV q6h **OR**

-Cefuroxime (Zinacef) 1.5 gm IV q8h **OR**
-Cefotaxime (Claforan) 1-2 gm IV q8 **OR**
-Ceftriaxone (Rocephin) 1-2 gm IV q12h **OR**
-Trimethoprim/Sulfamethoxazole (Septra DS) 6-10 mg TMP/kg/d IV in 2-3 divided doses **OR**
-Ampicillin/Sulbactam (Unasyn) 1.5 gm IV q6h.

COPD with pneumonia:
-Erythromycin 500 mg IV q6h **AND/OR**
-Cefuroxime axetil (Ceftin) 250-500 mg PO bid **OR**
-Cefotaxime (Claforan) 1-2 gm IV q4-6h **OR**
-Ceftriaxone (Rocephin) 1-2 gm IV q12h **OR**
-Ceftizoxime (Cefizox) 1-2 gm IV q8-12h **OR**
-Cefuroxime (Zinacef) 0.75-1.5 gm IV q8h **OR**
-Ampicillin/sulbactam (Unasyn) 1.5-3 gm IV q6h **OR**
-Amoxicillin/clavulanate (Augmentin) 250-500 mg PO q8h **OR**
-Ticarcillin/clavulanate (Timentin) 3.1 gm IV q4-6h (200-300 mg/kg/d).

Alcoholics, Diabetics, Heart Failure, Debilitated or other Underlying Diseases:
-Erythromycin 0.5-1.0 gm IV q6h **AND EITHER**
Cefotaxime (Claforan) 1-2 gm IV q4-6h **OR**
Ceftriaxone (Rocephin) 1-2 gm IV q12h **OR**
Cefuroxime (Zinacef) 0.75-1.5 gm IV q8h **OR**
Ceftizoxime (Cefizox) 1-2 gm IV q8 **OR**
TMP/SMX IV 6-10 mg TMP/Kg per day in 2-3 divided doses **OR**
Ampicillin/Sulbactam (Unasyn) 1.5-3 gm IV q6h. **OR**
Ticarcillin/clavulanate Timentin 3.1 gm IV q4-6h (200-300 mg/Kg/day).

Nosocomial, Hospital Acquired, Broad Spectrum Antibiotics Associated Pneumonia:
-Tobramycin 80-100 mg IV q8h (3-5 mg/kg/d) **AND EITHER**
Ceftriaxone 1-2 gm IV q12-24h **OR**
Ceftizoxime (Cefizox) or other 3rd generation cephalosporin (see above) **OR**
Piperacillin, Azlocillin, Mezlocillin or Ticarcillin 3 gm IV q4-6h (with tobramycin or gentamicin) **OR**
Imipenem/cilastatin (Primaxin) 0.5-1.0 gm IV q6-8h.

Aspiration Pneumonia (community acquired):
-Clindamycin (Cleocin) 600-900 mg IV q8h (with or without gentamicin or 3rd gen cephalosporin) **OR**
-Penicillin G 1-2 MU IV q4h (with or without gentamicin and/or 3rd gen cephalosporin) **OR**
-Ampicillin/Sulbactam (Unasyn) 1.5-3 gm IV q6h (with or without gentamicin or 3rd gen cephalosporin).
-Ticarcillin/Clavulanic acid (Timentin) 3.1 gm IV q4-6h (with or without Gentamicin) **OR**
-Imipenem/Cilastatin (Primaxin) 0.5-1.0 gm IV q6-8h

Aspiration Pneumonia (nosocomial):
-Tobramycin 2 mg/kg IV then 1.7 mg/kg IV q8h **OR**
-Ceftazidime 1-2 gm IV q8h **AND EITHER**
Clindamycin (Cleocin) 600-900 mg IV q8h **OR**

Penicillin G 1-2 MU IV q4h **OR**

Ampicillin/Sulbactam or Ticarcillin/clavulanate, or Imipenem/cilastatin (see above).

10. Symptomatic Medications:
   -Acetaminophen (Tylenol) 650 mg 2 tab PO q3-4h prn temp >101 or pain.
   -Docusate sodium (Colace) 100-200 mg PO qhs.
   -Ranitidine (Zantac) 150 mg PO bid.
   -Prochlorperazine (Compazine) 5-10 mg IV/PO q4-6h or 25 mg PR bid.

11. Extras: CXR PA, LAT, ECG, PPD.

12. Labs: CBC with diff, SMA 7 & 12, ABG. Blood C&S x 2. Sputum gram stain, C&S. Methenamine silver sputum stain (PCP); AFB smear/culture; fungal prep (KOH). Aminoglycoside levels peak & trough at 3rd dose. UA.
Cold agglutinins, acute/convalescent titers for chlamydia pneumonia (TWAR) mycoplasma, legionella, coccidiomycosis, skin tests (tuberculosis/coccidiomycosis mucositis) if indicated.

13. Other Orders and Meds:

___

SPECIFIC THERAPY OF PNEUMONIA

Pneumococcal pneumoniae Pneumonia:
   -Penicillin G 1-2 million units IV q4h **OR**
   -Erythromycin 500 mg IV q6h.

Staphylococcus aureus Pneumonia:
   -Oxacillin or Nafcillin 2 gm IV q4h **OR**
   -Vancomycin 500 mg IV q6h or 1 gm IV q12h (1 gm in 250 cc D5W over 1h q12h).

Klebsiella pneumoniae Pneumonia:
   -Gentamicin 1.5-2 mg/Kg IV, then 1.0-1.5 mg/Kg IV q8h (adjust for Azotemia). **AND EITHER**
   Ceftriaxone (Rocephin) 2 gm IV q12h **OR**
   Ceftizoxime (Cefizox) 1-2 gm IV q8h **OR**
   Ceftazidime (Fortaz) 1-2 gm IV q8h.

Haemophilus influenzae:
   -Ampicillin 1-2 gm IV q6h (ß-lactamase negative) **OR**
   -Cefuroxime 0.75-1.5 gm IV q8h (ß-lactamase pos) **OR**
   -Ceftizoxime (Cefizox) 1-2 gm IV q8h **OR**
   -Chloramphenicol 0.5-1.0 gm IV q6h.

Pseudomonas aeruginosa:
   -Tobramycin 1.5-2.0 mg/Kg IV, then 1.5-2.0 mg/Kg IV q8h (adjust for Azotemia) **AND EITHER**
   Piperacillin, Ticarcillin, Mezlocillin or Azlocillin 3 gm IV q4h **OR**
   Ceftazidime 1-2 gm IV q8h.

Mycoplasma pneumoniae:
-Clarithromycin (Biaxin) 250-500 mg PO bid 7-10 days **OR**
-Azithromycin (Zithromax) 500 mg PO x 1, then 250 mg PO qd x 4 days (T½ 60 hours). **OR**
-Erythromycin 500 mg PO or IV q6h x 14-21 days **OR**
-Tetracycline 250-500 mg PO q6h x 14-21 days.

Legionella pneumoniae:
-Erythromycin 1.0 gm IV q6h x 21 days **AND**
 Rifampin 600 mg PO qd x 21 days (if progression of disease on erythromycin; or alternate to erythromycin if intolerant).

Moraxella (Branhamella) catarrhalis:
-Ampicillin/sulbactam (Unasyn) 1.5-3 gm IV q6h **OR**
-Cefuroxime 0.75-1.5 gm IV q8h **OR**
-Erythromycin 0.5-1.0 gm IV q6h x 21 days **OR**
-Trimethoprim/SMX 160/800 mg DS IV q8-12h (6-10 mg TMP/kg/d)

Anaerobic Pneumonia:
-Penicillin G 1-2 MU IV q4h **OR**
-Clindamycin (Cleocin) 600-900 mg IV q8h. **OR**
-Metronidazole (Flagyl) 500 mg IV q6-8h.

13. Other Orders and Meds:

PNEUMOCYSTIS CARINII PNEUMONIA IN AIDS

1. Admit to:
2. Diagnosis: PCP pneumonia
3. Condition:
4. Vital signs: q2h; Call MD if BP >160/90, <90/60; P >120, <50; R>25, <10; T>38.5°C; 02 sat <90%
5. Activity:
6. Nursing: Weight qOD, pulse oximeter.
7. Diet: Regular, encourage fluids.
8. IV Fluids: D5½NS at 50-100 cc/h or TKO.
9. Special Medications:

PNEUMOCYSTIS CARINII PNEUMONIA:
-Trimethoprim/sulfamethoxazole (Bactrim, Septra) 15-20 mg/Kg/day (based on TMP) PO or IV in 3-4 divided doses x 21 days; and prednisone (if room air $PO_2 \leq 70$ mmHg or Aa gradient ≥ 35 mmHg) 40 mg PO bid x 5 days, then 20 mg PO bid x 5 days, then 20 mg PO qd x 11 days; or methylprednisolone 40 mg IV q8h. TMP-SMX is the drug of choice. **OR**
-Pentamidine (Pentam) 4 mg/Kg IV qd x 21 days, and Prednisone or Prednisolone as above. Pentamidine is alternate treatment if inadequate response to TMP-SMX. **OR**
-Dapsone (DDS) 100 mg PO qd x 21 days; and trimethoprim (Proloprim) 5 mg/Kg PO qid x 21 days (avoid dapsone if G-6-PD deficient **OR**

-Atovaquone (Mepron) 750 mg PO tid x 21 days. Use restricted to those with mild to moderate PCP who are refractory to or intolerant of TMP-SMX. **OR**

-Primaquine phosphate 15 mg base PO qd x 21 days; and clindamycin 600 mg IV q6h, or 300-450 mg PO qid x 21 days (avoid primaquine if G-6-PD deficient). **OR**

-Trimetrexate 45 mg/m² IV qd x 21 days; and folinic acid 20 mg/m² PO or IV q6h x 21 days.

PCP prophylaxis (previous PCP, CD4 <200)

-TMP/SMX DS (160/800 mg) PO qd or 3 times per week **OR**

-Pentamidine, 300 mg in 6 ml sterile water via Respirgard II nebulizer over 20-30 min q4 weeks; may pretreat with Albuterol 2.5 mg in 5 mL NS **OR**

-Dapsone (DDS) 50 mg PO qd or 100 mg PO twice weekly, avoid dapsone if G-6-PD deficient.

Anti HIV Therapy:

-Zidovudine (Retrovir)(CD4 <200, AIDS, advanced ARC) 200 mg po tid, or 500 mg po per day divided tid. Some authors hold anti-HIV therapy during TMP/SMX therapy because of the marrow suppressing side effects of both drugs combined **OR**

-Didanosine (DDI, Videx) 125-300 mg PO bid **OR**

-Zalcitabine (DDC, Hivid) 0.75 mg PO tid.

-Recombinant erythropoietin (Epogen, EPO) 100 U/Kg 3 times/wk to treat zidovudine-induced anemia if endogenous serum erythropoietin level ≤ 500 IU/L.

-**Post-exposure Prophylaxis**: Zidovudine, 200 mg PO q4h x 72h, then 100-200 mg 5 times/day x 25 days.

Zidovudine-Induced Neutropenia/Ganciclovir-Induced Leucopenia

-Recombinant human granulocyte colony-stimulating factor (G-CSF, generic name "Filgrastim", trade name "Neupogen") 1-2 mcg/Kg SQ qd until absolute neutrophil count 500-1000.

10. Other Medications:

-Ranitidine (Zantac) 150 mg PO bid or 50 mg IV q8h.

11. Extras: CXR PA & LAT. Gallium Scan if indicated; PFT's, diffusing capacity.

12. Labs: ABG, CBC, SMA 7 & 12, LDH (fractionated). Blood C&S x 2 for bacterial, fungal. Sputum for Gram stain, C&S, AFB. Giemsa (Diff-Quik), immunofluorescence, or silver stain for pneumocystis, fungal C&S. Induce sputum with nebulized 3% saline after gargling with 3% saline.

Serum CD4, CD8 lymphocyte count, VDRL, serum cryptococcal antigen, HBsAg, anti-HBs, titers for toxoplasmosis, sulfadiazine levels. UA.

Bronchoscopic Considerations: Consider bronchoscopic diagnosis if sputum non-diagnostic or CXR not typical for PCP or patient not responding to empiric therapy.

13. Other Orders and Meds:

OPPORTUNISTIC INFECTIONS IN AIDS

Oral Candidiasis:
-Clotrimazole (Mycelex) troches, 10 mg dissolved in mouth over 15-30 minutes, 3-5 times a day for 2 weeks **OR**
-Nystatin (Mycostatin), oral pastilles (200,000 units), one to two dissolved slowly in mouth five times a day; or vaginal tablets (100,000 U), dissolved slowly in mouth three times a day **OR**
-Ketoconazole (Nizoral), 200 mg po qd for two weeks **OR**
-Fluconazole (Diflucan), 50-100 mg po qd.

Candida Esophagitis:
-Fluconazole, 100-200 mg po qd x 2-3 weeks **OR**
-Ketoconazole, 200-400 mg po qd x 2-3 weeks **OR**
-Amphotericin B 0.3 mg/Kg IV qd x 7 days.
-Maintenance with fluconazole (100 mg po qd) or ketoconazole (200 mg po qd) may be required.

Primary or Recurrent Mucocutaneous HSV
-Acyclovir (Zovirax), 200-400 mg po 5 times a day for 10 days, or 5 mg/kg IV q 8 hr OR In cases of acyclovir resistance, Foscarnet, 40 mg/kg IV q8h, via infusion pump only, for 21 days.
-Prophylaxis: Acyclovir (Zovirax) 400 mg PO bid or foscarnet as above.

Herpes Simplex Encephalitis:
-Acyclovir 10 mg/kg IV q8h x 10-21 days.

Herpes Varicella Zoster
-Acyclovir 10-12 mg/kg IV over 60 min q8h for 7-14 days **OR** 800 mg PO 5 times/d x 7-10 days.

Cytomegalovirus infections:
-Ganciclovir (Cytovene) 5 mg/Kg IV (100 mls D5W or NS over 60 min) q12h x 14-21 days for retinitis, colitis, esophagitis (concurrent use with zidovudine may increase hematological toxicity). **OR**
-Foscarnet (Foscavir) 5 mg/Kg IV q8h x 14-21 days.
-G-CSF or GM-CSF 2.5-5.0 mcg/Kg SQ qd to treat ganciclovir-induced neutropenia.

Suppressive Treatment:
-Ganciclovir 5 mg/Kg IV qd, or 6 mg/Kg 5 times/wk, or foscarnet 90-120 mg IV qd.

TOXOPLASMOSIS:
-Pyrimethamine 200 mg PO, then 50-100 mg PO qd; and sulfadiazine 1.0-1.5 Gms PO q6h; and folinic acid 5-10 mg PO qd. **OR**
-Pyrimethamine 200 mg PO, then 50-100 mg PO qd; and clindamycin 450 mg PO q6h or 600 mg IV q6h; and folinic acid 5-10 mg PO qd. **OR**
-Atovaquone (Mepron) 750 mg PO q6h.

Suppressive Treatment:
-Pyrimethamine 25-50 mg PO qd with or without sulfadiazine 0.5-1.0 Gm PO q6h; and folinic acid 5-10 mg PO qd. **OR**
-Pyrimethamine 50 mg PO qd; and clindamycin 300 mg PO q6h; and folinic acid 5-10 mg PO qd.

Cryptococcus Neoformans Meningitis:
-Amphotericin B 0.5-0.8 mg/kg/d IV qd, over 4h x 8-12 weeks or until total dose of 2.0-2.5 gm. **AND**
Flucytosine (Ancobon) 25-37.5 mg/kg PO q6h x 4-6 weeks (decrease dose in renal failure, maintain peak levels <120 mg/L)

Suppressive Treatment:
-Fluconazole (Diflucan) 200 mg PO qd indefinitely.

Active Tuberculosis:
-Isoniazid (INH) 300 mg PO qd; and rifampin 600 mg PO qd; and pyrazin-amide 15-25 mg/Kg PO qd; and ethambutol 15-25 mg/Kg PO qd; or streptomycin 15 mg/Kg IM qd, or 20 mg/Kg IM twice/wk.
-Pyridoxine (Vitamin B6) 50 mg PO qd concurrent with INH.
-Multidrug treatment should continue for 6 months after cultures become negative.

Prophylaxis:
-Isoniazid 300 mg PO qd; and pyridoxine 50 mg PO qd x 12 months or longer.

DISSEMINATED MYCOBACTERIUM AVIUM COMPLEX (MAC):
-Clarithromycin (Biaxin) 500-1000 mg PO bid; or Azithromycin (Zithromax) 500 mg PO qd; **AND EITHER**
Ethambutol 15-25 mg/Kg PO qd, **OR**
Clofazimine (Lamprene) 100-200 mg PO qd, **OR**
Ciprofloxacin (Cipro) 750 mg PO bid or 400 mg IV bid.
-Some patients may not require treatment other patients may require indefinite treatment.

Prophylaxis:
-Rifabutin (Ansamycin) 300 mg PO qd or 150 mg PO bid.

DISSEMINATED COCCIDIOIDOMYCOSIS:
-Amphotericin B 0.5-0.8 mg/kg IV qd, until total dose 2.0-2.5 gms. **OR**
-Fluconazole (Diflucan) 400-800 mg PO and/or IV qd.

DISSEMINATED HISTOPLASMOSIS:
-Amphotericin B 0.5-0.8 mg/kg IV qd, until total dose 15 mg/kg. **OR**
-Itraconazole (Sporanox) 200 mg PO bid.
-AIDS associated diarrhea - see page 62

Suppressive Treatment:
-Itraconazole (Sporanox) 200 mg PO bid **OR**
-Amphotericin B 0.5-0.8 mg/Kg IV q/wk.

Other Orders and Meds:

SEPTIC ARTHRITIS

1. **Admit to:**
2. **Diagnosis:** Septic arthritis
3. **Condition:**
4. **Vital signs:** q shift
5. **Activity:** No weight bearing on infected joint. BSC
6. **Nursing:** Warm compresses prn, keep joint immobilized.
7. **Diet:** Regular
8. **IV Fluids:** D5W TKO
9. **Special Medications:**

Empiric Therapy for Adults without Gonorrhea contact:
-Nafcillin or Oxacillin 2 gm IV q4h **AND**
 Gentamicin 100-120 mg (1.5-2 mg/kg) IV, then 80 mg IV q8h (3-5 mg/kg/d)
 OR
-Vancomycin 500 mg IV q6h or 1 gm q12h (1 gm in 250 cc D5W over 60 min
 q12h) and Gentamicin as above **OR**
-Ticarcillin/clavulanate (Timentin) 3.1 gms IV q4-6h **OR**
-Ampicillin/Sulbactam (Unasyn) 1.5-3.0 gm IV q6h **OR**
-Imipenem/cilastatin (Primaxin) 0.5-1.0 gm IV q6-8h.

Empiric Therapy for Adults with possible Gonorrhea:
-Ceftriaxone (Rocephin) 1-2 gm IV q12h (max 4 gm/d) **OR**
-Spectinomycin 2 gm IM **OR**
-Ciprofloxacin (Cipro) 400 mg IV q12h.

Neisseria Gonorrhea:
-Ceftriaxone 1 gm IV qd x 7-10 days **OR**
-Ceftizoxime or cefotaxime, 1 gm IV q8h x 2-3 d or until improved, then
 cefuroxime axetil, 500 mg PO bid to complete 7-10 days of treatment.

Staphylococcus aureus:
-Nafcillin 1-2 gm IV q4h **OR**
-Vancomycin 1 gm IV q12h.

Staphylococcus epidermidis:
-Vancomycin 1 gm IV q12h.

Hemophilus influenza:
-Ampicillin (lactamase negative) 1-2 gms q4h **OR**
-Cefuroxime (lactamase positive) 1.5 gms IV q8h **OR**
-Ampicilliin/Sulbactam (Lactamase positive) 1.5-3.0 Gms IV q6h.

Streptococcus, Eikenella corrodens, Pasteurella multocida or Peptostreptococcus:
-Penicillin G 250,000 U/kg/d IV given in 6 divided doses.

Enterobacteriaceae (E coli, Klebsiella, Enterobacter, Salmonella):
-Cefotaxime (or other 3rd gen cephalosporin) 2 gm IV q6h x 21 days. **OR**
-Ampicillin 1-2 gm IV q4h x 2-3 days, then 1-1.5 gm PO q6h **OR**
-Trimethoprim/sulfamethoxazole DS 160/800 mg, 1-2 tabs PO bid x 14 days.

10. **Symptomatic Medications:**
-Acetaminophen & codeine (Tylenol 3) 1-2 PO q4-6h prn pain.
-Heparin 5000 U SQ bid.

11. Extras: X-ray views of joint, CXR, ECG, technetium/gallium scan, CT. Synovial biopsy & culture. PPD

12. Labs: CBC, SMA 7&12, ESR, blood C&S x 2, VDRL. UA. Cultures of urethra, cervix, urine, throat, sputum, skin, rectum. Antibiotic levels.

Synovial fluid:

> **Tube 1** - Glucose, protein, lactate, pH.
>
> **Tube 2** - Gram stain, C&S, fungal, AFB, CIE for H flu, meningococcus, strep pneumoniae.
>
> **Tube 3** - Cell count, light & polarizing crystals.

13. Other Orders and Meds:

SEPTIC SHOCK

1. Admit to:

2. Diagnosis: Sepsis

3. Condition:

4. Vital signs: q1h; Call MD if BP syst >160/90, <90/60; P >120, <50; R>25, <10; T>38.5°C; urine output < 25 cc/hr for 4h 02 saturation <90%.

5. Activity: Bed rest with bedside commode.

6. Nursing: I&O, pulse oximeter. Foley to closed drainage.

7. Diet: NPO

8. IV Fluids:

9. Special Medications:

  -Oxygen at 2-5 L/min by NC or mask.

Non-immunocompromised Adults. Antibiotics: if pelvic or intra-abdominal infection, use ampicillin or vancomycin with gent/tobra, add clindamycin or metronidazole ; **OR** use cefoxitin & gent/tobra **OR** Unasyn & gent/tobra. May use 3rd generation cephalosporins in place of aminoglycosides if resistant gram-neg pathogens not suspected.

  -Ceftazidime (Fortaz) 1-2 g IV q8h **OR**

  -Ceftizoxime (Cefizox) 1-2 gm IV q8h **OR**

  -Cefotaxime (Claforan) 2 gm q4-6h **OR**

  -Ceftriaxone (Rocephin) 1-2 gm IV q12h (max 4 gm/d). **OR**

  -Cefoxitin (Mefoxin) 1-2 gms IV q6-8h **OR**

  -Cefotetan (Cefotan) 1-2 Gms IV q12h **OR**

  -Cefotetan (Cefotan) 1-2 Gms IV q12h **OR**

  -Ampicillin 2 gm IV q4h **OR**

  -Piperacillin, ticarcillin or mezlocillin 3 gms IV q4-6h **AND**

  -Gentamicin or tobramycin 100-120 mg (1.5-2 mg/kg) IV, then 80 mg IV q8h (3-5 mg/kg/d) **AND**

  -Clindamycin 600-900 IV q8h (15-30 mg/kg/d) **OR**

  -Metronidazole 500 mg (7.5 gm/kg) IV q6h **OR**

  -Ticarcillin/clavulanic acid (Timentin) 3.1 gm IV q4-6h (200-300 mg/kg/d) (with gent/tobra). **OR**

  -Ampicillin/Sulbactam (Unasyn) 1.5-3.0 gm IV q6h (with gent/tobra) **OR**

  -Imipenem/cilastatin (Primaxin) 0.5-1.0 gm IV q6-8h (with gent/tobra).

-Vancomycin 500 mg IV q6h or 1 gm IV q12h.

Nosocomial sepsis with IV catheter or IV drug abuse

-Vancomycin 500 mg IV q6h or 1 gm q12h (1 gm in 250 cc D5W over 60 min q12h); **AND**

Gentamicin or Tobramycin as above; **AND EITHER**

Ceftazidime or Ceftizoxime 1-2 gms IV q8h **OR**

Piperacillin, ticarcillin or mezlocillin 3 gm IV q4-6h.

Blood Pressure Support

-Dopamine 4-20 µg/kg/min (200 mg in 250 cc D5W, 800 µg/ml).

-Albumin 25 gm IV (100 ml of 25% sln) **OR**

-Hetastarch (Hespan) 500-1000 cc over 30-60 min (max 1500 cc/d).

-Dobutamine (tissue oxygenation support; use in addition to agents need for BP support) 5 mcg/kg/min, and titrate up to max 15 mcg/kg/min to get maximum increase in cardiac index, and oxygen transport without decreasing mean arterial pressure; goal is to improve SVO_2.

CANDIDA SEPTICEMIA:

-Amphotericin B, 1mg test dose (D5W 100mls 60 min), then 10-20 mg (D5W 250 mls over 3-4h) the sme day, then 0.4-0.5 mg/Kg/day (D5W 250-500 mls over 4-6h); total dose 0.5-1.0 gm.

10. Symptomatic Medications:

-Acetaminophen 650 mg PR 30 min prior to Ampho B

-Diphenhydramine 25-50 mg IV 30 min prior to Ampho B

-Meperidine 25-50 mg IV prn shaking/chills during Ampho B infusion

-Ranitidine (Zantac) 50 mg IV q8h or 150 mg PO bid.

-Heparin 5000 units SQ q8-12h.

11. Extras: CXR, KUB, sinus films, ECG, Indium/Gallium scan, ultrasound, lumbar puncture. Cardiology consult or critical care consult consider Swan Ganz placement, especially in setting of left ventricular failure).

12. Labs: CBC with diff, SMA 7 & 12, blood C&S x 3, Gram stain of buffy coat blood, T&C for 3-6 Units PRBC, PT/PTT, fibrinogen, FDP, thrombin time, gent levels peak & trough at 3rd dose. UA with micro. Cultures of urine, sputum, wound, IV catheters, ascitic fluid, decubitus ulcers, pleural fluid.

13. Other Orders and Meds:

PERITONITIS

1. Admit to:

2. Diagnosis: Peritonitis

3. Condition:

4. Vital signs: q1h; Call MD if BP >160/90, <90/60; P >120, <50; R>25, <10; T>38.5°C

5. Activity: Bed rest with legs elevated, bedside commode.

6. Nursing: Guaiac all stools.

7. Diet: NPO

8. IV Fluids: D5½ NS, 20 mEq KCL/L at 125 cc/h

9. Special Medications:
Spontaneous Bacterial Peritonitis (nephrotic or cirrhotic):
Option 1:
   -Ampicillin * 1-2 gms IV q 4-6h; **AND EITHER**
   Cefotaxime (Claforan) 1-2 gm IV q4-6h **OR**
   Ceftizoxime (Cefizox) 1-2 gms IV q8h **OR**
   Gentamicin or Tobramycin 1.5 mg/Kg IV, then 1 mg/Kg q8h (adjust for renal function).

Option 2:
   -Ticarcillin/clavulanate (Timentin) 3.1 gms IV q6h.

Option 3:
   -Imipenem/cilastatin (Primaxin) 0.5-1.0 gm IV q6h.

*Vancomycin 500 mg IV q6h or 1 gm IV q12h if penicillin allergic.

Secondary Bacterial Peritonitis:
Option 1:
   -Cefoxitin (Mefoxin) 2 gm IV q6-8h **OR**
   -Ampicillin 1-2 gm IV q4-6h **AND**
   Gentamicin or tobramycin (aminoglycosides are not recommended in cirrhotics) 100-120 mg (1.5 mg/kg); then 80 mg IV q8h (5 mg/kg/d)(if resistant, use amikacin) **AND**
   Metronidazole 500 mg IV q6h (15-30 mg/kg/d)

Option 2:
   -Ticarcillin/clavulanic acid (Timentin) 3.1 gm IV q4-6h (200-300 mg/kg/d) with aminoglycoside as above.

Option 3:
   -Ampicillin/Sulbactam (Unasyn) 1.5-3.0 gm IV q6h with aminoglycoside as above.

Option 4:
   -Imipenem/cilastatin (Primaxin) 0.5-1.0 gm IV q6-8h.

Peritonitis Associated with Ambulatory Peritoneal Dialysis:
   -Tobramycin 70-140 mg/2 L bag initially then 8-16 mg/2 L maintenance **AND/OR**
   -Vancomycin 1000-1200 mg/2 L initially then 30-50 mg/2 L maintenance.
   #### Fungal:
   -Amphotericin B (2 mg/L 1st 24 hours then 1.5 mg/L) **AND**
   Flucytosine (100 mg/L 1st 3 days then 30 mg/L)

10. Symptomatic Meds:
   -Ranitidine (Zantac) 50 mg IV q8h or 150 mg PO bid.
   -Acetaminophen 325 mg PO q4-6h prn temp >101.

11. Extras: plain film, upright abdomen, lateral decubitus, CXR PA & LAT; stat surgery consult for secondary bacterial peritonitis; ECG, abdominal ultrasound, Indium/Gallium scan. CT scan abdomen/pelvis with contrast

12. Labs: CBC with diff, SMA 7 & 12, albumin, LDH, amylase, lactate. PT/PTT, UA with micro, C&S; gent levels peak & trough at 3rd dose.

PARACENTESIS TUBE 1 - Cell count & differential (1-2 ml, EDTA purple top tube)

TUBE 2 - Gram stain of sediment, C&S, AFB, fungal C&S (3-4 ml); inject 10-20 ml into anaerobic & aerobic culture bottle.

TUBE 3 - Glucose, protein, albumin, LDH, triglycerides, specific gravity, bilirubin, amylase, fibrinogen, fibronectin (2-3 ml, red top tube).

SYRINGE - pH, lactate (3 ml).

13. Other Orders and Meds:

DIVERTICULITIS

1. **Admit to:**
2. **Diagnosis:** Diverticulitis
3. **Condition:**
4. **Vital signs:** qid; Call MD if BP syst >160/90, <90/60; P >120, <50; R>25, <10; T>38.5°C
5. **Activity:** Up ad lib in room.
6. **Nursing:** Daily weights, I&O. Guaiac all stools.
7. **Diet:** NPO
8. **IV Fluids:** 0.5-2 L NS over 1-2hr then, D5½NS with 20 mEq KCL at 125 cc/hr. Cantor or Miller-Abbot intestinal tube or 10-18 F Levin NG tube at low intermittent suction (if obstructed).
9. **Special Medications:**

Regimen 1:
-Gentamicin or tobramycin 100-120 mg IV (1.5-2 mg/kg), then 80 mg IV tid (5 mg/kg/d) **AND EITHER**
Cefoxitin (Mefoxin) 2 gm IV q6-8h **OR**
Clindamycin (Cleocin) 600-900 mg IV q8h.

Regimen 2:
-Metronidazole 1 g (15 mg/kg) IV then 500 mg q6-8h (15-30 mg/kg/d) **AND**
Ciprofloxacin (Cipro) 250-500 mg PO bid or 200-300 mg IV q12h

Outpatient Regimen:
-Trimethoprim/SMX (Bactrim DS) 160/800 mg DS PO bid (and clindamycin or metronidazole PO)

10. **Symptomatic Medications:**
-Ranitidine (Zantac) 50 mg IV q8h or 150 mg PO bid.
-Meperidine 50-100 mg IM or IV q3-4h prn pain.
11. **Extras:** Acute abdomen series, CXR PA & LAT, ECG, low pressure gastrografin enema, surgery and GI consults. CT scan with contrast
12. **Labs:** CBC with diff, SMA 7 & 12, amylase, lipase, blood cultures x 2, gent levels peak & trough at 3rd dose. UA with micro, C&S.
13. **Other Orders and Meds:**

LOWER URINARY TRACT INFECTION

1. **Admit to:**
2. **Diagnosis:** UTI
3. **Condition:**
4. **Vital signs:** tid; Call MD if BP <90/60; >160/90; R >30, <10; P >120, <50; T>38.5°C
5. **Activity:**
6. **Nursing:**
7. **Diet:** Regular
8. **IV Fluids:**
9. **Special Medications:**

<u>**Lower Urinary Tract Infection:**</u>
 -Trimethoprim/SMX (Septra) 2 double strength tabs PO x 1 dose or 160/800 mg PO bid x 3-10 d **OR**
 -Amoxicillin/clavulanate (Augmentin) 250 mg or 500 mg tab PO bid-tid **OR**
 -Nitrofurantoin (Macrodantin) 100 mg PO q6h **OR**
 -Norfloxacin (Noroxin) 400 mg PO bid x 3-10 d **OR**
 -Ciprofloxacin (Cipro) 250 mg PO bid x 3-10 d or 200 mg IV q12h **OR**
 -Cephalothin (Keflex) 500 mg PO q6h **OR**
 -Cefixime (Suprax) 200 mg PO q12h or 400 mg PO qd **OR**
 -Cefazolin (Ancef) 1-2 gm IV q8h.
 -Amoxicillin (in pregnancy) 500 mg PO q8h 3-10 d.

<u>**Complicated or Catheter Associated Urinary Tract Infection:**</u>
 -Ampicillin 1 gm IV q4-6h **AND EITHER**
 Cefazolin (Ancef) 1-2 gm IV q8h **OR**
 Ceftizoxime (Ceftizox) 1 gm IV q8h. **OR**
 Ceftriaxone (Rocephin) 0.5-1 gm IV q12h **OR**
 Aztreonam (Azactam) 1-2 gm IV q6-8h **OR**
 Gentamicin 100-120 mg IV (1.5-2 mg/kg); then 80 mg IV q8h (1.5/kg q8-12h) **OR**
 -Ticarcillin/clavulanic acid (Timentin) 3.1 gm IV q4-6h
 -Ciprofloxacin or Norfloxacin (see above).

<u>**Prophylaxis ($\geq$ 3 episodes/yr):**</u>
 -Trimethoprim/SMX ½ single strength tab PO qd (after eradication of infection).

CANDIDA CYSTITIS
 -Amphotericin B continuous bladder irrigation, 50 mg/1000 ml sterile water (50 µg/ml) via 3-way foley catheter at 1 L/d for 5 days **OR**
 -Fluconazole (Diflucan) 100 mg PO or IV x 1 dose, then 50 mg PO or IV qd for 5 days.

10. **Symptomatic Medications:**
 -Phenazopyridine (Pyridium) 100-200 mg PO tid.
11. **Extras:** Renal ultrasound, IVP, postvoid residual volume.
12. **Labs:** CBC, SMA 7. UA with micro, urine Gram stain, C&S.
13. **Other Orders and Meds:**

PYELONEPHRITIS

1. **Admit to:**
2. **Diagnosis:** Pyelonephritis
3. **Condition:**
4. **Vital signs:** tid; Call MD if BP <90/60; >160/90; R >30, <10; P >120, <50; T>38.5°C
5. **Activity:**
6. **Nursing:** I&O, daily weights
7. **Diet:** Regular
8. **IV Fluids:** D5½ NS with 20 mEq KCL at 100 cc/h.
9. **Special Medications:**
   -Ampicillin* 1 gm IV q4-6h **AND EITHER**
   Gentamicin or tobramycin - loading dose of 100-120 mg IV (1.5-2 mg/kg); then 80 mg IV q8h (2-5 mg/kg/d) **OR**
   Ceftizoxime (Cefizox) 1 gm IV q8h **OR**
   Ceftazidime (Fortaz) 1 gm IV q8h.
   -Ticarcillin/clavulanate (Timentin) 3.1 gm IV q6h
   -Imipenem/cilastatin (Primaxin) 0.5-1.0 gm q6-8h.
   -Ciprofloxacin (Cipro) 250-500 mg PO bid or 200 mg IV q12h.
   -Norfloxacin (Noroxin) 400 mg PO bid.
   -Amoxicillin/clavulanate (Augmentin) 250 mg or 500 mg tab PO tid
   -Trimethoprim/SMX (TMP-SMX, Septra) 160/800 mg (1 DS tab) PO bid or IV (10 mls in 100 mls D5W over 2h) q12h
   -*Use vancomycin if allergic to penicillin 500 mg IV q6h or 1 gm IV q12h.
10. **Symptomatic Medications:**
    -Phenazopyridine (Pyridium) 100-200 mg PO tid.
    -Meperidine (Demerol) 25-100 mg IM q4-6h prn pain.
11. **Extras:** Renal ultrasound, IVP, postvoid residual volume, KUB.
12. **Labs:** CBC with diff, SMA 7. UA with micro, urine Gram stain, C&S, blood C&S x 2. Vancomycin & gent levels peak & trough at 3rd or 4th dose.
13. **Other Orders and Meds:**

OSTEOMYELITIS

1. **Admit to:**
2. **Diagnosis:** Osteomyelitis
3. **Condition:**
4. **Vital signs:** qid; Call MD if BP <90/60; T>38.5°C
5. **Activity:**
6. **Nursing:** Keep involved extremity elevated.
7. **Diet:** Regular, high fiber.
8. **IV Fluids:** Hep-lock with flush q shift.

9. Special Medications:

Adult Empiric Therapy (staph a. gram neg. strep):
  -Nafcillin or Oxacillin 2 gm IV q4h
  -Cefazolin (Ancef) 1-2 gm IV q8h
  -Vancomycin 500 mg q6h or 1 gm q12h (1 gm in 250 cc D5W over 1h q12h)
  -**Add** 3rd generation cephalosporin if gram negative bacilli on Gram stain.
    Treat for 4-6 weeks

Post Operative or Post trauma (staph a. gram neg. Pseudomonas):
  -Vancomycin 500 mg IV q6h or 1 gm q12h **AND** Ceftazidime (Fortaz) 1-2 gm
    IV q8h.
  -Imipenem/cilastatin (Primaxin)**(single drug Tx)** 0.5-1.0 gm IV q6-8h.
  -Ticarcillin/clavulanic acid (Timentin)**(single drug Tx)** 3.1 gm IV q4-6h (200-
    300 mg/kg/d).
  -Ciprofloxacin (Cipro) 500 mg PO bid or 200-300 mg IV q12h **AND**
    Rifampin 600 mg PO qd.
  -Treat for 4-6 weeks.

Osteomyelitis with Decubitus Ulcer:
  -Cefoxitin (Mefoxin) see above.
  -Ciprofloxacin (Cipro) and clindamycin or metronidazole.
  -Imipenem/cilastatin (Primaxin), see above.
  -Nafcillin, gentamicin and clindamycin; see above.
  -Treat for 4-6 weeks.

10. Symptomatic Medications:
  -Meperidine 50-100 mg IM q3-4h prn pain.
  -Docusate sodium (Colace) 100-200 mg PO qhs.
  -Heparin 5000 U SQ bid.

11. Extras: Technetium and Gallium bone scans, multiple X-ray views (mark ulcer with wire), CT/MRI, CXR PA & LAT.

12. Labs: CBC with diff, SMA 7, blood C&S x 3, MIC, MBC, UA with micro, C&S. Needle biopsy, antibiotic levels peak & trough at 3rd dose.

13. Other Orders and Meds:

TUBERCULOSIS
(Immunocompetent Host)

1. Admit to:

2. Diagnosis: Active Pulmonary Tuberculosis

3. Condition:

4. Vital signs: q shift

5. Activity: Up ad lib in room.

6. Nursing: Respiratory isolation for 1-2 weeks after starting Tx, collect all
  sputum.

7. Diet: Regular

8. Special Medications:
  -Isoniazid 300 mg PO qd (5 mg/kg/d, max 300 mg/d) for 6 months **AND**
  -Rifampin 600 mg PO qd (10 mg/kg/d, 600 mg/d max) for 6 months **AND**

-Pyrazinamide 1.5-2.0 gm (15-30 mg/kg/d, max 2 gm) PO qd for 6 months **AND**

-Ethambutol 1.5 gm (25 mg/kg/d, 2.5 gm/d max) PO qd **(if resistance to INH is likely)**.

Prophylaxis

-Isoniazid 300 mg PO qd (5 mg/kg/d) x 6 months (12 months if HIV positive).

9. Extras: CXR PA, LAT & lordotic views, spinal series, ECG.

10. Labs: CBC with diff, SMA7 & 12, LFT's, HIV. First AM sputum for AFB x 3 samples, then send sputum q2d. UA with micro, C&S, AFB.

11. Other Orders and Meds:

CELLULITIS

1. Admit to:

2. Diagnosis: Cellulitis

3. Condition:

4. Vital signs: tid; Call MD if BP <90/60; T>38.5°C

5. Activity: Up ad lib.

6. Nursing: Keep affected extremity elevated; warm compresses prn.

7. Diet: Regular, encourage fluids.

8. IV Fluids: Hep lock with flush q shift.

9. Special Medications:

Empiric Therapy Cellulitis

-Nafcillin or Oxacillin 1-2 gm IV q4-6h.

-Cefazolin (Ancef) 1-2 gm IV q8h.

-Vancomycin 500 mg IV q6h or 1 gm q12h (1 gm in 250 cc D5W over 1h q12h).

-Dicloxacillin 250-500 mg PO qid (in mild disease or after improvement on IV therapy).

-Penicillin (only if high suspicion of erysipelas) 1-1.5 million U IV q4h (2-6 MU/d).

Immunosuppressed, Diabetic Patients or Ulcerated Lesions:

-Use Nafcillin or cefazolin + (gent or aztreonam + clindamycin or metronidazole if septic) **OR** Timentin **OR** Imipenem **OR** Cipro + clindamycin or metronidazole.

-Nafcillin or oxacillin 1-2 gm IV q4-6h.

-Cefazolin (Ancef) 1-2 gm IV q8h.

-Cefoxitin (Mefoxin) 1-2 gm IV q6-8h.

If Septic: Gentamicin 100-120 mg IV (1.5-3 mg/kg), then 80 mg IV q8h (3-5 mg/kg/d) **OR** Aztreonam (Azactam) 1-2 gm IV q6-8h **PLUS**

-Clindamycin (Cleocin) 600-900 mg IV q8h or 450 mg PO qid **OR**

-Metronidazole (Flagyl) 500 mg IV/PO q6h.

-Ticarcillin/clavulanic acid (Timentin) **(single drug Tx)** 3.1 gm IV q4-6h (200-300 mg/kg/d).

-Ampicillin/Sulbactam (Unasyn)**(single drug therapy)** 1.5-3.0 gm IV q6h.

-Imipenem/cilastatin (Primaxin)**(single drug therapy)** 0.5-1 mg IV q6-8h **OR**

-Ciprofloxacin (Cipro) 250-500 mg PO bid or 200-300 mg IV q12h **AND**
Clindamycin 250-500 mg PO bid or 600-900 mg IV q8h (or metronidazole).

Necrotizing Soft-tissue Infection
-Penicillin 3-4 million Units IV q4h **AND**
Gentamicin (see above) **AND EITHER**
Metronidazole 1 g (15 mg/kg) IV over 1h, then 500 mg (7.5 mg/kg) q6h **OR**
Clindamycin (Cleocin) 600-900 mg IV q8h.

10. Symptomatic Medications:
-Silver sulfadiazine or ½ strength Dakin's sln wet to dry dressings tid. 1:1000
Betadine soaks qd.
-Tylenol #3 PO q4h prn pain **OR**
-Codeine 30 mg PO q4-6h prn pain.

11. Extras: X-ray views of site, Technetium/Gallium scans, doppler analysis
(ankle-brachial indices), impedance plethysmography, bone biopsy.

12. Labs: CBC, SMA 7, blood C&S x 2. Leading edge aspirate, swab, drainage
fluid for Gram stain, C&S, UA, antibiotic levels.

13. Other Orders and Meds:

PELVIC INFLAMMATORY DISEASE

1. Admit to:

2. Diagnosis: Pelvic Inflammatory Disease

3. Condition:

4. Vital signs: q4h x 24h then qid; Call MD if BP >160/90, <90/60; P >120,
<50; R>25, <10; T>38.5°C

5. Activity:

6. Nursing: I&O, qOD weights.

7. Diet: Regular

8. IV Fluids: D5½NS at 100 cc/hr.

9. Special Medications:
-Cefoxitin (Mefoxin) 2 gm IV q6h **OR** Cefotetan (Cefotan) 1-2 gms IV q12h;
AND
Doxycycline (Vibramycin) 100 mg IV q12h (IV for 4 days & 48h after
afebrile, then complete 10-14 days of Doxycycline 100 mg PO bid)
-Gentamicin 100-120 mg (2 mg/kg), then 100 mg (1.5 mg/kg) IV q8h **AND**
Clindamycin 900 mg IV q8h, then complete 10-14 d of Clindamycin 450 mg
PO qid or Doxycycline 100 mg PO bid.

10. Symptomatic Medications:
-Triazolam (Halcion) 0.125-0.5 mg PO qhs prn sleep.
-Acetaminophen 325 mg 1-2 tabs PO q4-6h prn pain or temp >101.
-Meperidine (Demerol) 25-100 mg IM q4-6h prn pain.

11. Labs: CBC, SMA 7 & 12, ESR. GC & chlamydia culture, gent levels. UA
with micro, C&S, VDRL, pregnancy test. Pelvic ultrasound.

12. Other Orders and Meds:

NEUTROPENIC FEVER, ONCOLOGIC EMERGENCY
(PMN's <1000)

1. Admit to:

2. Diagnosis: Neutropenic fever

3. Condition:

4. Vital Signs: q2-4h: call M.D. if BP <90/60; >160/90; R>30 <10; P 7/20 <50; T >38.5° <36.0°

5. Activity: Bedrest with BRP

6. Nursing: I/O, daily weights; change IV catheter/change Foley catheter: Send catheter tips for culture and Gram stain; strict reverse isolation; no flowers or plants at bedside.

7. Diet: Neutropenic precautions: no vegetable matter.

8. IVF: D5½NS with 20 mcg KCL/L at 30 cc/h.

9. Special Medications:
-Ceftazidime 2 gm IV q8h **OR**
-Piperacillin **OR** Mezlocillin 3-4 gm IV q4h **AND**
 Gentamicin **OR** Tobramycin 2 mg/kg loading dose followed by 1.5 mg/kg q8h (adjust for renal disease) **AND**
-Vancomycin 500 mg IV q6h (if staphylococcus infection is suspected) **AND**
-Clindamycin 900 mg IV q8h (if mucositis or periodontal infection present).
   CONSIDER
-Amphotericin B 0.5-0.7 mg/kg IV qd (after test dose) if persistent fever after 5-7 days on broad spectrum antibiotics, consider empiric treatment for candida sepsis.

10. Symptomatic meds:
-Meperidine (Demerol) 25-100 mg IM/IV q4-6h prn pain.
-Diphenhydramine (Benadryl) 25-50 mg PO qhs prn insomnia.
-Mild of magnesia 30 cc PO q12h prn constipation.

11. Extras:
-If indwelling central catheter, consider discontinuing and send for Gram stain, C&S; biopsy cutaneous lesions; thoracentesis, paracentesis, lumbar puncture, infectious disease consult.

12. Labs:
CBC with diff, SMA7/12, PT/PTT; UA with micro; C&S/Gram stain.
Oral, skin, soft tissue lesions - Gram stain, C&S, fungal culture, viral culture. Stool - C&S, ova & parasites x 3; Wright's stain; CXR, consider decubitus films; blood cultures (aerobic/anaerobic/fungal) x 3. C. difficile toxin assay (if diarrhea due to recent antibiotic use).

13. Other Orders/Meds:
-Nystatin susp/Benadryl/antacid/lidocaine (vicious) mixture with 5% sodium bicarbonate soln swish/spit q2-4h (prophylactic/therapeutic mouth care in mucositis).
-Vitamin K 10 mg SQ x 3 (if ↑ PT due to prolonged antibiotic use).

GASTROENTEROLOGY

PEPTIC ULCER DISEASE

1. **Admit to:**
2. **Diagnosis:** Duodenal/gastric ulcer
3. **Condition:**
4. **Vital signs:** qid, postural BP; Call MD if BP syst >160, <90; diast. >90, <60; P >120, <50; T>38.5°C
5. **Activity:** Up ad lib
6. **Nursing:** Guaiac all stools.
7. **Diet:** NPO 48h, then regular, no caffeine.
8. **IV Fluids:** D5½NS with 20 mEq KCL at 125 cc/h. Levin 10-18 F NG tube at low intermittent suction (if obstructed).
9. **Special Medications:**
   -Ranitidine (Zantac) 50 mg IV bolus, then continuous infusion at 6.25-12.5 mg/h (150-300 mg in 500 ml D5W at 21 ml/h over 24h) or 50 mg IV q8h, or 150 mg PO bid or 300 mg PO qhs.
   -Cimetidine (Tagamet) 300 mg IV bolus, then continuous infusion at 37.5-50 mg/h (900 mg in 500 ml D5W over 24h) or 300 mg IV q6-8h, or 300 mg PO qid or 400 mg PO bid or 800 mg PO qhs.
   -Famotidine (Pepcid) 20 mg IV q12h or 40 mg PO qhs or 20 mg PO bid.
   -Nizatidine (Axid) 300 mg PO qhs or 150 mg PO bid.
   -Sucralfate (Carafate)**(not with H2 blockers or if scheduled for endoscopy)** 1 gm PO qid or 2 gm PO bid (1/2 h ac & hs, may dissolve in 10 ml water).
   -Omeprazole (Prilosec) 20-40 mg PO qd, maximum 8 weeks.
   -GI cocktail - Mylanta 30 cc, Donnatal 10 cc, viscous lidocaine 5-10 cc PO.
10. **Symptomatic Medications:**
    -Trimethobenzamide (Tigan) 100-250 mg PO or 100-200 mg IM/PR q6h prn nausea **OR**
    -Prochlorperazine (Compazine) 5-10 mg IM/IV/PO q4-6h, or 25 mg PR q4-6h prn nausea.
    -Codeine sulfate 30 mg PO q4-6h prn pain **OR**
    -Meperidine (Demerol) 50-100 mg IM q3-4h prn pain **OR**
    -Morphine Sulfate infusion 0.03-0.05 mg/kg/h continuous IV infusion (50-100 mg in 500 ml D5W) titrated to pain.
11. **Extras:** Upright abdomen, KUB, CXR, ECG, upper GI series, endoscopy, GI consult. Surgery consult.
12. **Labs:** CBC, SMA 7 & 12, calcium, amylase, lipase, LDH. UA, fasting serum gastrin qAM x 3 day (hypersecretory syndrome); secretin stimulation test (antral G cell hyperplasia). Salicylate level, cyclooxygenase level
13. **Other Orders and Meds:**

GASTROINTESTINAL BLEEDING

1. **Admit to:**
2. **Diagnosis:** Upper/lower GI bleed
3. **Condition:**
4. **Vital signs:** q30min; Call MD if BP >160/90, <90/60; P >120, <50; R>25, <10; T>38.5°C; urine output <25 ml/hr for 4h; CVP >15; orthostatic vitals bid.
5. **Activity:** Bed rest
6. **Nursing:** Place 32-36 F Ewald tube or 18 F Salem-sump (double lumen) or 18 F Levin (single lumen) NG tube, then lavage with 2 L of room temperature NS, then connect low intermittent suction, repeat lavage q1h. Record volume & character of lavage; consider removal of NG tube when bleed not active. Foley to closed drainage; I&O; NG aspirate q2h for pH & gastrocult; keep gastric pH > 4 with 10-80 cc Mylanta. Record stool character. Pulse oximeter.
7. **Diet:** NPO
8. **IV Fluids:** Two 16 gauge IV lines. 3 L NS over 1-4h; when available, transfuse 2-6 units PRBC run as fast as possible, then call MD for further orders.
9. **Special Medications:**
   -Oxygen 2-5 L by NC.
   -Ranitidine (Zantac) 50 mg IV bolus, then continuous infusion at 6.25-12.5 mg/h [150-300 mg in 500 ml D5W over 24h (21 cc/h)], or 50 mg IV q6-8h, followed by 150 mg PO bid **OR**
   -Cimetidine (Tagamet) 300 mg IV bolus, then continuous infusion at 37.5-50 mg/h (900 mg in 500 cc D5W over 24h), or 300 mg IV q6-8h, followed by 300 mg PO tid-qid **OR**
   -Famotidine (Pepcid) 20 mg IV q12h, followed by 20 mg PO q12h **OR**
   -Omeprazole (Prilosec) 20-40 mg PO qd.

   <u>Suspected Esophageal Variceal Bleeds:</u>
   -Vasopressin (Pitressin) 20 U IV over 20-30 minutes, then 0.2-0.3 U/min [100 U in 250 ml of D5W (0.4 U/ml)], for 30 min, followed by increases of 0.2 U/min until bleeding stops or max of 0.9 U/min. If bleeding stops, taper over 24-48h **AND**
   -Nitropaste (with vasopressin) 1 inch q6h **OR** nitroglycerin IV at 10-30 mcg/min continuous infusion (50 mg in 250 mls D5W) (lessens vasoconstriction of peripheral vessels)
   -Vitamin K (Phytonadione, Aquamephyton) 10 mg IV/SQ qd for 3 days (continue only if PT↑).
   -Fresh frozen plasma 2-4 U IV (in severe coagulopathies or after 6-8 U PRBC).

10. **Extras:** Potable CXR, upright abdomen, ECG. Surgery & GI consults.
   <u>Upper GI Bleeds:</u> Esophagogastroduodenoscopy with possible coagulation or sclerotherapy; Sengstaken-Blakemore or Minnesota tube for tamponade (usually requires intubation).
   <u>Lower GI Bleeds:</u> Sigmoidoscopy/colonoscopy, (after a Golytely purge 6-8 L over 4-6h) technecium 99m RBC scan, angiography with possible embolization.
11. **Labs:** CBC, platelets, SMA 7 & 12, SGPT, SGOT, GGT, alkaline phosphatase, LDH, bilirubin, lactate, salicylate level, PT/PTT, type and cross for 3-6 U PRBC & 2-4 U FFP. Spun hematocrit q4h with CBC q12-24h.

12. Other Orders and Meds:

___

CIRRHOTIC ASCITES & EDEMA

1. **Admit to:**
2. **Diagnosis:** Cirrhotic ascites & edema
3. **Condition:**
4. **Vital signs:** Vitals, neurochecks & urine output qid; Call MD if BP >160/90, <90/60; P >120, <50; T>38.5°C; urine output < 25 cc/hr x 4h, or abnormal mental status.
5. **Activity:** Bed rest with legs elevated.
6. **Nursing:** I&O, daily weights, measure abdominal girth qd, guaiac all stools.
7. **Diet:** 250-500 mg sodium/d, protein intake 60 gm/d (with alcoholic hepatitis, severe hepatic insufficiency or shunt: 1.5 gm/kg protein); fluid restriction to 1-1.5 L/d (if hyponatremia, Na <130).
8. **IV Fluids:** Hep-lock with flush q shift.
9. **Special Medications:**
   -Diurese to reduce weight by 0.5-1 kg/d (if edema) or 0.25 kg/d (if no edema). Discontinue hepatotoxic drugs: aldomet, isoniazid, nitrofurantoin.
   -Spironolactone (Aldactone) 25-50 mg PO qid or 200 mg PO qAM, increase by 100 mg/d to max of 400 mg/d.
   -Amiloride 5 mg PO qd, increase by 5 mg/d to max 40 mg PO qd.
   -Furosemide (Lasix)(ascites refractory to above) 40-120 mg PO or IV qd-bid.
   -Hydrochlorothiazide 50-100 mg PO qd.
   -KCl 20-40 mEq PO qAM (use with lasix).
   -Metolazone (Zaroxolyn) 5-20 mg PO qd.
   -Captopril (resistant ascites) 12.5-25 mg PO q8h.
   -Ranitidine (Zantac) 150 mg PO bid.
   -Cimetidine (Tagamet) 300 mg PO tid-qid.
   -Vitamin K 10 mg SQ qd x 3d.
   -Folic acid 1 mg PO qd.
   -Thiamine 100 mg PO qd.
   -Multivitamin PO qd.

   Paracentesis: remove up to 5 L ascites if peripheral edema, tense ascites, or ↓ diaphragmatic excursion. If large volume paracentesis give salt-poor albumin 12.5 gm with each L of paracentesis fluid removed (50 ml of 25% solution); infuse 25 ml before paracentesis menadiol 10 mg IV over 60 min qd or & 25 ml 6h after.

Also see Hepatic Encephalopathy, page 68.

10. **Symptomatic Medications:**
    -Docusate sodium (Colace) 100-200 mg PO qhs.
11. **Extras:** KUB, CXR, abdominal ultrasound, doppler flow studies of portal vasculature, 99mTc-liver spleen scan, GI consult. Consider liver biopsy if unclear etiology without significant coagulopathy and after resolution ascites.
12. **Labs:** Ammonia, CBC, SMA 7 & 12, LFT's, albumin, LDH, SGGT, 5'-nucleotidase, amylase, lipase, blood C&S, PT/PTT, bleeding time, blood alcohol,

plasma oncotic pressure. Urine Cr, Na, K. Repeat SMA7, urine creatinine & Na qAM.

Ferritin, TIBC (hemochromatosis), ceruloplasmin, urine copper (Wilson's disease) HBsAg, HBc IgM, anti-HBc Ag, anti-HBsAg/IgG, HBeAg or H_B DNA), anti HC, HDV RNA, anti-delta (IgM/IgG)(viral hepatitis) alpha-1-antitrypsin, ANA, anti-smooth muscle Ab, soluble liver/kidney microsomal Ab, serum electrophoresis (autoimmune hepatitis) antimitochondrial Ab (primary biliary cirrhosis).

Ascitic Fluid

Tube 1 - protein, albumin, specific gravity, glucose, bilirubin, amylase, lipase, triglyceride, LDH, fibrinogen, fibronectin (3-5 ml, red top tube).

Tube 2 - Cell count & differential (3-5 ml, purple top tube).

Tube 3 - C&S, Gram stain, AFB, fungal (5-20 ml); inject 20 ml into blood culture bottles. At bedside.

Tube 4 - Cytology (>20 ml).

Syringe - pH (2 ml).

Concomitant serum albumin, LDH, total protein, glucose.

13. Other Orders and Meds:

VIRAL HEPATITIS

1. Admit to:

2. Diagnosis: Hepatitis

3. Condition:

4. Vital signs: qid; Call MD if BP <90/60; T>38.5°C

5. Activity:

6. Nursing: Stool Isolation, guaiac all stools.

7. Diet: Clear liquid (if nausea), Low fat (if diarrhea), 2 gm salt (edema or ascites), protein intake of 40 gm/d, increase at 10 gm increments q2d as tolerated until 100 gm/d (1.5 g/kg/d).

8. Special Medications:
   -Cimetidine (Tagamet) 300 mg PO tid-qid **OR**
   -Sucralfate 1 gm PO qid (1h ac & hs).
   -Vitamin K 10 mg SQ qd x 3d.
   -Multivitamin PO qd.
   -HAV immune globulin (Gamastan)(for contacts) 0.02 ml/kg IM.
   -Hepatitis B immune globulin 0.06 ml/kg IM left deltoid, for fluid & blood contacts within 2 weeks exposure **AND**
   -HBV vaccine (Recombivax-B, Heptavax, Engerix-B) (for contacts) 1 ml IM/SQ right deltoid, repeat in 1 & 6 months.
   -Discontinue hepatotoxic medications: methyldopa, isoniazid, nitrofurantoin.

9. Symptomatic Meds:
   -Meperidine (Demerol) 25-100 mg IM q4-6h prn pain.
   -Prochlorperazine (Compazine) 5-10 mg PO/IM q4-6h prn.
   -Hydroxyzine (Vistaril) 25 mg IM/PO q4-6h prn nausea or pruritus.
   -Diphenhydramine (Benadryl) 25-50 mg PO/IV q4-6h prn pruritus or sleep.

10. Extras: Liver/spleen scan, ultrasound, GI consult; consider liver biopsy if uncertain etiology without significant coagulopathy or ascites.

11. Labs: CBC, SMA 7 & 12, SGGT, LDH, 5'-nucleotidase, amylase, lipase, PT/PTT; acetaminophen level, anti-HA IgM, HBsAg, anti-HBc (IgM/IgG), HBeAg, HCAb, anti-HBe, anti-HBs, HDV-RNA, anti-delta (IgM/IgG); hep E serology (if available); Monospot, EBV titer, herpes titer, CMV titer (viral hepatitis); alpha 1 antitrypsin level. ANA, anti-smooth muscle Ab, soluble liver/kidney microsomal Ab. Ferritin, TIBC, ceruloplasmin; urine copper.

12. Other Orders and Meds:

CHOLECYSTITIS

1. Admit to:

2. Diagnosis: Cholecystitis

3. Condition:

4. Vital signs: q4h; call MD if BP >160/90, <90/60; P>120, <50; R>25, <10; T>38.5°C

5. Activity: Bed rest with bedside commode.

6. Nursing: Daily weights, I&O.

7. Diet: NPO

8. IV Fluids: 0.5-2 L LR over 1-2h then D5½NS with 20 mEq KCl/L at 125 cc/hr. Levin NG tube (10-18 F) at low constant suction.

9. Special Medications:
  -Metronidazole 1.0 gm (15 mg/kg) over 1h, then 500 mg (7.5 mg/kg) IV q6h
  AND EITHER
  Mezlocillin, Azlocillin or Piperacillin 3 gm IV q4-6h **or**
  Cefoxitin (Mefoxin) 1-2 gm IV q6-8h **or**
  Cefotetan (Cefotan) 1-2 gm IV q12h.
  -Imipenem Cilastatin 0.5-1.0 gm IV q6h (single drug treatment).
  -Ampicillin/Sulbactam (Unasyn)**(single drug Tx)** 1.5-3 gm IV q6h.
  -Ticarcillin/Clavulanate (Timentin) **(single drug Tx)** 3.1 g IV q4-6h.   In seriously ill patient consider adding aminoglycoside.

10. Symptomatic Medications:
  -Meperidine 50-100 mg IM q4-6h prn pain **OR**
  -Pentazocine (Talwin) 30-60 mg IM q3-4h.

11. Extras: Upper abdomen ultrasound, HIDA scan, CXR PA & LAT, KUB, ECG. Surgical consult; GI consult for possible ERCP if choledocholithiasis.

12. Labs: CBC, SMA 7 & 12, GGT, LDH, amylase, lipase, PT/PTT, hepatitis panel, type & hold 2 U PRBC. UA.

13. Other Orders and Meds:

BACTERIAL CHOLANGITIS & BILIARY SEPSIS

1. **Admit to:**
2. **Diagnosis:** Bacterial cholangitis
3. **Condition:**
4. **Vital signs:** q1h; Call MD if BP syst >160, <90; diast. >90, <60; P >120, <50; R>25, <10; T>38.5°C
5. **Activity:** Bed rest
6. **Nursing:** I&O
7. **Diet:** NPO
8. **IV Fluids:** 0.5-3 L LR over 1-3h, then D5½NS with 20 mEq KCl/L at 125 cc/h. Levin NG tube (10-18 F) at low constant suction. Foley to closed drainage.
9. **Special Medications:**
   -Mezlocillin, Azlocillin or Piperacillin 3 gm IV q4-6h **AND**
   Metronidazole (Flagyl) 500 mg (7.5 mg/kg) IV q6h.
   -Cefoxitin (Mefoxin) 1-2 gm IV q6-8h (with gentamicin).
   -Ticarcillin/clavulanate (Timentin) 3.1 g IV q4-6h.
   -Ampicillin 1-2 gm IV q4-6h. **AND**
   Gentamicin 100 mg (1.5-2 mg/kg), then 80 mg IV q8h (3-5 mg/kg/d) **AND**
   Metronidazole 500 mg (7.5 mg/kg) IV q6h .
10. **Symptomatic Medications:**
    -Meperidine (Demerol) 25-100 mg IM q4-6h prn pain.
11. **Extras:** CXR, ECG, RUQ & liver ultrasound (rule out liver abscess), HIDA, acute abdomen series. GI consult (possible ERCP and sphincterotomy).
12. **Labs:** CBC, SMA 7 & 12, GGT, LDH, amylase, lipase, blood C&S x 2. UA, PT/PTT, gentamicin levels peak & trough at 4th dose.
13. **Other Orders and Meds:**

ACUTE PANCREATITIS

1. **Admit to:**
2. **Diagnosis:** Acute pancreatitis
3. **Condition:**
4. **Vital signs:** q1h, orthostatic vitals bid; Call MD if BP >160/90, <90/60; P >120, <50; R>25, <10; T>38.5°C; urine output < 25 cc/hr.
5. **Activity:** Bed rest with bedside commode.
6. **Nursing:** Daily weights, I&O, fingerstick glucose qid, guaiac stools.
7. **Diet:** NPO
8. **IV Fluids:** 1-4 L NS over 1-3h, then D5½NS with 20 mEq KCl/L at 125 cc/hr. 10-18 F Levin NG tube at low constant suction (if obstruction); aspirate q2h for pH & gastrocult; keep pH >4 with 10-80 cc Mylanta. Foley to closed drainage.
9. **Special Medications:**
   -Ranitidine (Zantac) 6.25-12.5 mg/h (0.2-0.4 mg/kg/h)(150- 300 mg in 500 ml D5W at 21 ml/h) IV or 50 mg IV q6-8h.
   -Cimetidine (Tagamet) 37.5-100 mg/h IV or 300 mg IV q6-8h.

-Famotidine (Pepcid) 20 mg IV q12h.
-Albumin 25 gm IV (100 ml of 25% solution) or 250 ml 5% sln.
-Antibiotics not required in uncomplicated pancreatitis. If suspicion of sepsis, rule out infected pseudocyst/ abscess with CT scan guided aspiration.
-Cefoxitin (Mefoxin) 1-2 gm IV q6-8h
-Heparin 5000 U SQ q12h.
-Total Parenteral Nutrition, if malnutrition or inability to tolerate orals for >3-5 days; see page 66.

10. Symptomatic Medications:
-Meperidine 50-100 mg IM q3-4h prn pain.

11. Extras: Upright abdomen, portable CXR for tube placement, ECG, ultrasound, Gastrografin upper GI, CT with contrast, Indium scan. Surgery and GI consult.

12. Labs: CBC, platelets, SMA 7 & 12, ionized & total calcium, triglycerides, amylase, lipase, LDH, SGOT, GGT, ABG, blood C&S x 2, coagulation panel, HBsAg, PT/PTT, type & hold 4-6 U PRBC & 2-4 U FFP. Pancreatic isoamylase, immunoreactive trypsin, chymotrypsin, elastase, CA 19-9 antigen. UA, urinary amylase & CR.

13. Other Orders and Meds:

EMPIRIC THERAPY OF DIARRHEA

1. Admit to:

2. Diagnosis: Diarrhea

3. Condition:

4. Vital signs: q4h; postural BP & Temp tid; Call MD if BP >160/90, <80/60; P>120; R>25; T>38.5°C

5. Activity: Up ad lib in room if no postural BP changes.

6. Nursing: Daily weights, I&O, stool volumes, urine specific gravity each void. NG at low intermittent suction if obstruction or other complication.

7. Diet: NPO except ice chips x 24h, then low residual elemental diet; no milk products; consider parenteral nutrition if severely malnourished.

8. IV Fluids: 1-3 L NS over 1-3 hours; then D5½NS with 40 mEq KCl/L at 150 cc/h.

9. Special Medications: antibiotics indicated only if toxic (fever, gross blood in stool, neutrophils) or after culture results with indications.

Febrile or gross blood in stool or neutrophils on microscopic exam or prior travel to subtropics or tropics:
-Ciprofloxacin (Cipro) 250-500 mg PO bid x 10-14 days **OR**
-Norfloxacin (Noroxin) 400 mg PO bid **OR**
-Trimethoprim/SMX (Bactrim DS) one double strength (160/800 mg) tab PO bid x 10-14 days.

Symptomatic Meds if indicated:
-Kaopectate 60-90 cc PO qid or after each loose BM prn **OR**
-Loperamide (Imodium) 2-4 mg PO tid-qid prn, max 16 mg/d **OR**
-Pepto Bismol 30 cc PO q30min x 8 hours.

-Diphenoxylate HCL (Lomotil) 1-2 tabs PO qid, max 12 tabs/day.

11. Extras: upright abdomen, CXR PA & LAT. GI consult for unprepared sigmoidoscopy/colonoscopy with biopsy/culture. Possible upper GI barium study; barium enema, ultrasound (liver/RUQ, rule out abscess)

12. Labs: SMA7 & 12, CBC with diff, UA, PT/PTT, blood culture x 2. Amebic serum titers, HIV test.

Stool studies: Wright's stain, ova & parasites x 3, C difficile toxin & culture, C&S (Yersinia, Campylobacter, Neisseria (GC), Shigella, Salmonella, Vibrio, Isospora, Cryptosporidium, Escherichia coli 0157:H7)

Osmotic diarrhea: stool/serum osmolality, stool anion gap, pH, stool phenolphthalein test, 24 hour fecal fat collection with standard diet. Reducing substances, pH.

Special tests for malabsorption syndrome: Schilling test (4-part), hydrogen breath test, D-xylose test, bile acid breath test, bentiromide test, lactose tolerance test. Upper GI with SBFT, EGD with small bowel biopsy.

Secretory diarrhea: stool/plasma osmolality; stool cultures, vasoactive intestinal polypeptide, 5 HIAA (systemic mastocytosis) calcitonin, serotonin, fasting serum gastrin level (Zollinger-Ellison); stool phenolphthalein test, consider malabsorption workup.

13. Other Orders & Meds: Discontinue medications if possible cause of diarrhea: laxatives, antacids, lactulose, colchicine, quinidine, enteral feedings, misoprostol, ampicillin, clindamycin.

SPECIFIC THERAPY OF DIARRHEA

AIDS ASSOCIATED DIARRHEA (severe refractory secretory diarrhea):
-Octreotide (Sandostatin) 200-300 mcg SQ in 2-4 divided doses x 2 weeks.

Shigella Sonnei:
-Ampicillin (susceptible strains) 500 mg PO qid x 3-5 days **OR**

-Trimethoprim/SMX, (Bactrim) double strength tab PO bid x 3-5 days **OR**

-Ciprofloxacin 500 mg PO bid x 5 day (best in patient's allergic to sulfa).

Salmonella (bacteremia):
-Bactrim DS PO/IV bid x 14 days **OR**

-Ampicillin 2 gms IV q6h x 14 days **OR**

-Chloramphenicol 500-1000 mg IV q6h x 14 days **OR**

-Ceftriaxone 1-2 gms IV q12h x 14 days. **OR**

-Ciprofloxacin 500 mg PO bid x 14 days.

Campylobacter jejuni:
-Erythromycin 250 mg PO qid x 5-10 days **OR**

-Ciprofloxacin 500 mg PO bid x 5-10 days.

Enterotoxic/Enteroinvasive E coli (Travelers Diarrhea):
-Trimethoprim/SMX (Bactrim), double strength tab PO bid x 5-7 days **OR**

-Ciprofloxacin 500 mg PO bid x 5-7 days.

ANTIBIOTIC ASSOCIATED & PSEUDOMEMBRANOUS COLITIS: (Clostridium difficile)(discontinue offending antibiotic):
-Metronidazole (Flagyl) 250 mg PO or IV qid x 10-14 days **OR**
-Vancomycin 125 mg PO qid x 10 days (500 PO qid x 10-14 days, if recurrent).

Vibrio (Cholera/Parahaemolyticus):
-Tetracycline 500 mg PO qid x 5-7 days **OR**
-Ciprofloxacin 500 mg PO bid x 5-7 days.

Yersinia Enterocolitica (sepsis):
-Gentamicin 1.5 mg/kg IV load, then 1 mg/kg IV q8h x 5-7 days, peak & trough level at 3rd dose **OR**
-Trimethoprim/SMX (Bactrim), double strength tab PO bid x 5-7 days **OR**
-Ciprofloxacin 500 mg PO bid x 5-7 days.

Cytomegalovirus Colitis/Viral (rarely indicated unless AIDS patient):
-Ganciclovir 5 mg/kg IV q12h x 14 days.

Entamoeba Histolytica (Amebiasis):
Asymptomatic cyst carrier:
-Iodoquinol 650 mg PO tid x 20 days **OR**
-Paromomycin 25-30 mg/kg/d in 3 doses x 7 days **OR**
-Diloxanide sulfate 500 mg PO tid x 10 days.
Mild to moderate intestinal disease:
-Metronidazole (Flagyl) 750 mg PO tid x 10 days **OR**
-Tinidazole 2 gm per day PO x 3 days. **Followed By:**
-Iodoquinol 650 mg PO tid x 20 days **OR**
-Paromomycin 25-30 mg/kg/d PO in 3 divided doses x 7 days.
Severe intestinal disease:
-Metronidazole 750 mg PO tid x 10 days **OR**
-Tinidazole 600 mg PO bid x 5 days **Followed By:**
-Iodoquinol 650 mg PO tid x 20 days **OR**
-Paromomycin 25-30 mg/kg/d PO in 3 divided doses x 7 days.

Giardia Lamblia:
-Quinacrine HCl 100 mg PO tid x 5d **OR**
-Metronidazole 250 mg PO tid x 7 days.

Isospora Belli:
-Trimethoprim/SMX (Bactrim), 4 single strength tabs PO bid x 2-3 weeks.

Cryptosporidium:
-Spiramycin 1 gm PO tid (investigational).

Other Orders & Meds:

___

ULCERATIVE COLITIS & CROHN'S DISEASE

1. **Admit to:**
2. **Diagnosis:** Ulcerative colitis/Crohn's disease.
3. **Condition:**
4. **Vital signs:** q4h, postural BP & temp tid; Call MD if BP >160/90, <90/60; P >120, <50; R>25, <10; T>38.5°C
5. **Activity:** Up ad lib in room.
6. **Nursing:** Daily weights, I&O. NG at low intermittent suction (if obstruction or other complications).
7. **Diet:** NPO except for ice chips x 48h, then low residue or elemental diet, no milk products.
8. **IV Fluids:** 1-3 L NS over 1-3h, then D5 1/2 NS with 40 mEq KCL/L at 150 cc/hr.
9. **Special Medications:**

Ulcerative colitis
   -Sulfasalazine (Azulfidine) 0.5-1 gm PO bid, increase over 10 d as tolerated to 0.5-1.0 gm PO qid **OR**
   -Olsalazine (Dipentum) 500 mg PO bid **OR**
   -5-aminosalicylate enema (Mesalamine) 4 gm/60 ml PR qhs (retain for 8h)(left colitis) **OR**
   -Hydrocortisone 50-100 mg IV q6h **OR**
   -Methylprednisolone 10-20 mg IV q6h **OR**
   -Prednisone 40-60 mg/d PO in divided doses.
   -6-mercaptopurine 50-100 mg PO qd or 2.0 mg/kg/d **OR**
   -Azathioprine 50-100 mg PO qd or 2 mg/kg/d.

Crohn's disease
   -NPO except for ice chips/medications for 48-72h, low fat, low oxalate, high calcium diet
   -Prednisone 40-60 mg/d PO in divided doses **OR**
   -Hydrocortisone 50-100 mg IV q6h.
   -Sulfasalazine (Azulfidine) 0.5-1 gm PO bid; increase over 10 d to 0.5-1 gm PO qid **OR**
   -Olsalazine (Dipentum) 500 mg PO bid **OR**
   -6-mercaptopurine 50-100 mg PO qd or 2.0 mg/kg/d **OR**
   -Azathioprine 50 mg PO bid (max 2 mg/kg/d)(chronic active disease).
   -Metronidazole 250 mg PO tid.

Other Medications:
   -B12, 100 µg IM x 5d then 100-200 µg IM q month.
   -Multivitamin PO qAM or 1 ampule IV qAM.
   -Folate 1 mg PO qd. (especially is sulfasalazine used)
   -FeSO4 300 mg PO qd-tid with meals.
   -Enteral (elemental) or Parenteral Nutrition, see page 66.

10. **Symptomatic Medications:**
   -Loperamide (Imodium) 2-4 mg PO tid-qid prn, max 16 mg/d (not in acute phase) **OR**
   -Kaopectate 60-90 ml PO qid prn.

11. Extras: Upright abdomen, UGI with SBFT, air contrast barium enema, CT scan abdomen/pelvis with contrast (Crohn's disease - rule out fistula/abscess, not in acute phase). Indium leukocyte scan & fecal excretion. CXR. PPD with controls, colonoscopy. Surgical & GI, dietetics consults.

12. Labs: CBC with diff & smear, platelets, SMA 7 & 12, Mg, ionized calcium, liver panel, blood C&S x 2, stool Wright's stain, stool amylase & lipase.

13. Other Orders and Meds:

PARENTERAL & ENTERAL NUTRITION

General Considerations: Daily weights, I&O. Nasoduodenal feeding tube or 10 F Cantor NG. HOB at 30° while enteral feeding & 2 hours after completion. Finger stick glucose qid, record bowel movements.

Enteral Bolus Feeding - Give 50-100 ml of enteral solution (Jevity, Vionex, Osmolite) q3h initially. Increase amount in 50 ml steps to max of 250-300 ml q3-4h; 30 kcal of nonprotein calories/kg/d & 1.5 gm protein/kg/d. Before each feeding measure residual volume, and delay feeding by 1h if >100 ml. Flush tube with 100 cc of water after each bolus.

Continuous enteral infusion - Initial enteral solution (Jevity, Vionex, Osmolite) 30 ml/hr. Measure residual volume q1h x 12h then tid; hold feeding for 1h if >100 ml. Increase rate by 25-50 ml/hr at 24 hr intervals as tolerated until final rate of 50-100 ml/hr as tolerated. 3 Tablespoonfuls of protein powder (Promix) may be added to each 500 cc of solution. Flush tube with 100 cc water q8h.

Peripheral Parenteral Supplementation:
- 3% amino acid sln (Procalamine) up to 3 L/d at 125 cc/h **OR**
- Combine 500 ml Amino acid solution 7% or 10% (Aminosyn) & 500 ml 20% dextrose & electrolyte additive and infuse at up to 100 cc/hr in parallel with:
- Intralipid 10% or 20% at 1 ml/min for 15 min (test dose); if no adverse reactions, infuse 500 ml/d at 21 mls/h over 24h, or up to 100 mls/h over 5 hours daily.
- Draw triglyceride level 6h after end of Intralipid infusion.

Central Parenteral Nutrition:
- Infuse 40-50 ml/h of amino acid-dextrose solution in the first 24h; increase daily by 40 ml/hr increments until providing 1.3-2 x basal energy requirement & 1.2-1.7 gm protein/kg/d (see formula page 96).

Standard solution:

Amino acid sln (Aminosyn) 7-10%	.500 ml
Dextrose 40-70%	.500 ml
Sodium	.35 mEq
Potassium	.36 mEq
Chloride	.35 mEq
Calcium	.4.5 mEq
Phosphate	.9 mmol
Magnesium	.8.0 mEq

Acetate . . . . .82-104 mEq
Multi-Trace Element Formula. . . . . .1 ml/d
  (Zn, copper, manganese, chromium)
Regular insulin (if indicated) . . . . .10-60 U/L
Multivitamin(12)(2 amp) . . . . .10 ml/d
  (vit C, A, D, E, B12, thiamine, riboflavin, pyridoxine,
  niacinamide, pantothenate, biotin, folate)
Vitamin K (in solution, SQ, IM) . . . . .10 mg/week
Vitamin B12. . . . . .1000 µg/week

WITH OR WITHOUT:

  Intralipid 20% 500 ml/d IVPB infuse in parallel with standard solution at 1 ml/min x 15 min; if no adverse reactions, increase to 100 ml/hr. Obtain serum triglyceride 6h after end of infusion (maintain <250 mg/dl).

  CYCLIC TPN 12h night schedule; Taper continuous infusion in morning by reducing rate to half original rate for 1 hour. Further reduce rate by half for an additional hr; then discontinue. Finger stick glucose q2h; Restart TPN in afternoon. Taper in beginning & end of cycle; Final rate of 185 ml/hr for 9-10h & 2h of taper at each end for total of 2000 ml.

7. Special Medications:
  -Metoclopramide (Reglan) 10-20 mg PO, IM, IV, or in J tube q6h.
  -Cimetidine 300 mg PO tid-qid or 37.5-100 mg/h IV or 300 mg IV q6-8h or in TPN **OR**
  -Ranitidine 50 mg IV q6-8h or 150 mg PO bid or in TPN.
  -Insulin sliding scale.

8. Symptomatic Medications:
  -Loperamide (Imodium) 2-4 mg PO/J-tube q6h, max 16 mg/d prn **OR**
  -Diphenoxylate/atropine (Lomotil) 1-2 tabs or 5-10 ml (2.5 mg/5 mls) PO/J-tube q4-6h prn, max 12 tabs/d **OR**
  -Codeine sulfate 30 mg PO or in J-tube q6h.
  -Kaopectate 30 cc PO or in J-tube q8h.

9. Extras: CXR, plain film for tube placement, Nutrition consult.

10. Labs:
  Baseline - draw all labs below.
  Daily labs - SMA7, osmolality, CBC, cholesterol, triglyceride (6 h after infusion), urine glucose & specific gravity.
  Twice weekly Labs - Cal, phosphatase, SMA-12
  Weekly Labs when indicated - Protein, Mg, iron, TIBC, transferrin, PT/PTT, zinc, copper, B12, Folate, 24h urine nitrogen & creatinine. Pre-albumin, retinol-binding protein.

11. Other Orders and Meds:

HEPATIC ENCEPHALOPATHY

1. **Admit to:**
2. **Diagnosis:** Hepatic encephalopathy
3. **Condition:**
4. **Vital signs:** q1h, neurochecks qid; Call MD if BP >160/90,<90/60; P >120,<50; R>25,<10; T>38.5°C
5. **Allergies:** Avoid sedatives, diuretics, NSAIDS or hepatotoxic drugs.
6. **Activity:** Bed rest.
7. **Nursing:** Keep HOB at 40 degrees, guaiac stools, turn patient q2h while awake, chart stools, notify MD if stool < 2/d. Seizure precautions, egg crate mattress, soft restraints prn.
8. **Diet:** Clear liquid x 24h, then 2100 Cal diet (25-40 Cal/kg/d), No protein x 48h then advance to 20-40 gm/d protein as tolerated, then increase in 20 gm increments q4d until adequate. Consider in patient unable to tolerate PO's with severe malnutrition and liver disease. Branched chain amino acids (HepatAmine) 500 ml with 500 ml 50% dextrose plus electrolytes & vitamins, infuse at 50-125 ml/h.
9. **IV Fluids:** D5W at TKO, Foley to closed drainage.
10. **Special Medications:**
    -Milk of magnesia 30 mg PO x 1 dose before starting lactulose.
    -Sodium biphosphate (Fleet) enema 118 ml PR x 1.
    -Lactulose 30-45 ml PO q1h x 3 doses, then 15-45 ml PO bid-qid titrate to produce 3 soft stools/d. **OR**
    -Lactulose enema 300 ml in 700 ml of tap water bid-qid, (may use rectal balloon catheter to retain 30-60 min, left side Trendelenburg x 15 min, then right side with head elevated) **AND**
    -Neomycin 1 gm PO q4-6h (4-12 g/d) **OR**
    -Metronidazole 250 mg PO q6h.
    -Ranitidine (Zantac) 50 mg IV q6-8h or 150 mg PO bid **OR**
    -Cimetidine (Tagamet) 37.5-50 mg/h IV or 300 mg IV q6-8h or 300 mg PO tid-qid **OR**
    -Famotidine (Pepcid) 20 mg IV/PO q12h
    -Vitamin K 10 mg SQ or IM qd x 3d.
    -Multivitamin PO qAM or 1 ampule IV qAM.
    -Folic acid 1 mg PO/IV qd.
    -Thiamine 100 mg PO/IV qd.
11. **Extras:** CXR, ECG, EEG, GI & dietetics consults.
12. **Labs:** Ammonia, CBC, platelets, SMA 7 & 12, Mg, Cal, SGOT, SGPT, SGGT, LDH, alkaline phosphatase, protein, albumin, bilirubin, 5'-nucleotidase, PT/PTT, ABG, blood C&S x 2, hepatitis panel. UA (1+ C&S) with micro, urine pH, electrolytes, Cr. Lumbar puncture (suspected meningitis). If ascites present, diagnostic paracentesis to rule out spontaneous bacterial peritonitis.
13. **Other Orders and Meds:**

ALCOHOL WITHDRAWAL

1. **Admit to:**
2. **Diagnosis:** Alcohol withdrawals / Delirium tremens.
3. **Condition:**
4. **Vital signs:** q4h; Call MD if BP >160/90, <90/60; P >130, <50; R>25, <10; T>38.5°C; or increase in agitation, or change neurological status.
5. **Activity:**
6. **Nursing:** Seizure & aspiration precautions, keep room well lit & quiet, guaiac stools, soft restraints prn.
7. **Diet:** Regular, push fluids.
8. **IV Fluids:** Hep-lock or D5½NS at 100-175 cc/h; multivitamin 1 amp qd; folate 1 mg qd; MgSO4 2-8 gm (to run in over 2-8h).
9. **Special Medications:**
   Withdrawal syndrome:
   -Chlordiazepoxide (Librium) 50-100 mg PO/IM/IV q6h x 3 days **OR**
   -Diazepam (Valium) 5-20 mg PO/IV q6-8h **OR**
   -Clonidine 0.1 mg PO qid , increase gradually to 0.2-0.4 mg qid.
   Delirium tremens:
   -Chlordiazepoxide 100 mg slow IV push or PO , repeat q4-6h prn agitation or tremor x 24h. Max 500 mg/d. Then give 50-100 mg PO q6h prn agitation or tremor **OR**
   -Diazepam (Valium) 5 mg IV repeat q6h until calm then 5-10 mg PO q4-6h.
   Seizures:
   -Diazepam 5-10 mg IV q5-15 min prn seizures, may repeat 5 mg q10-15min prn; max dose 30 mg. (chronic anticonvulsant therapy usually not indicated unless structural CNS disease).
10. **Symptomatic Medications:**
    -Magnesium sulfate 1 gm in 100 ml D5W over 2h qd.
    -Multivitamin 1 amp IV then 1 tab PO qd.
    -Folate 1 mg PO qd (if not given IV).
    -Thiamine 100 mg PO qd (if not given IV).
    -Haloperidol (Haldol) 1-5 mg PO tid or 2-5 mg IM/IV q3-4h prn severe agitation.
    -Acetaminophen 325-625 mg PO q4-6h prn headache. (Less than 3 gm qd).
    -Metoclopramide (Reglan) 10 mg PO, IV or IM q6h prn nausea.
11. **Extras:** CXR, ECG. Alcohol rehab & social work consult.
12. **Labs:** CBC, RBC indices, SMA 7 & 12, Mg, amylase, lipase, liver panel, VDRL, blood alcohol, urine drug screens. UA, PT/PTT.
13. **Other Orders and Meds:**

TOXICOLOGY

POISONING & DRUG OVERDOSE

DECONTAMINATION:

Ipecac (not if ingestion of acid/base, caustics, tricyclics, or if obtundent, impaired gag reflex, seizing):
- Ipecac syrup (<1h after ingestion), 30 ml with 240-480 ml liquid, may repeat x 1 after 30min if no emesis.

Gastric Lavage: Left side down, place catheter & check position by injecting air & auscultating. NS lavage until clear fluid, then leave activated charcoal or other antidote prn. Contraindicated in corrosives.

Cathartics:
- Magnesium Citrate 6% sln 150-300 ml PO
- Magnesium sulfate 10% solution 150-300 ml PO.

Activated Charcoal: 50 gm PO (first dose should be given using product containing sorbitol as cathartic). Repeat q2-6h if indicated.

Hemodialysis: Isopropanol, Methanol, Ethylene glycol, Severe salicylate intoxication (>100 mg/dl), lithium, theophylline (if neurotoxicity, seizures, or coma) with charcoal hypoperfusion.

ANTIDOTES:

NARCOTIC OR PROPOXYPHENE OVERDOSE:
- Naloxone hydrochloride (Narcan) 0.4 mg IV/ET/IM/SC/sublingual may repeat q2min.

METHANOL OR ETHYLENE GLYCOL OVERDOSE:
- Ethanol 60-80 ml (10% inj sln) IV over 30min, then 0.8-1.4 ml/kg/h. Maintain Ethanol level 100-150 mg/100 mL.

CARBON MONOXIDE OVERDOSE:
- Hyperbaric oxygen therapy or 100% oxygen by mask if HBO not available.

PHENOTHIAZINE OR EXTRAPYRAMIDAL REACTION:
- Diphenhydramine (Benadryl) 25-50 mg IV/IM q6h x 4 doses; followed by 25-50 mg IV/PO q6h for 24-72h prn **OR**
- Benztropine (Cogentin) 1-2 mg IV, then 1-2 mg IV/PO bid prn.

BENZODIAZEPINE OVERDOSE (Diazepam, Midazolam, Lorazepam, Alprazolam):
- Flumazenil (Romazicon) 0.2 mg (2 ml) IV over 30 sec q1 min until a total dose of 3 mg, if a partial response occurs, continue 0.5 mg increments until a total of 5 mg. If the patient has continued sedation (does not appreciably reverse respiratory depression), repeat the above regimen or start a continuous IV infusion 0.1-0.5 mg/h. Excessive doses, beyond reversal of sedation, may cause seizures.

Labs: Drug screen (serum, gastric, urine); blood levels, SMA 7, fingerstick glucose, CBC, ABG, ammonia, LFT's, ECG.

Other Orders and Meds:

ACETAMINOPHEN OVERDOSE

1. **Admit to:** Medical intensive care unit.
2. **Diagnosis:** Acetaminophen overdose
3. **Condition:**
4. **Vital signs:** q1h with neurochecks; Call MD if BP >160/90, <90/60; P >130, <50; R>25, <10; urine output <20 cc/h.
5. **Activity:** Bed rest with BSC.
6. **Nursing:** I&O, pulse oximeter, aspiration & seizure precautions, guaiac stools. Place large bore (Ewald) NG tube, then lavage with 2 L of NS.
7. **Diet:** NPO
8. **IV Fluids:**
9. **Special Medications:**
   -Ipecac syrup 30 cc PO.
   -Activated Charcoal 30-100 gm doses, remove via NG suction prior to acetylcysteine.
   -Acetylcysteine (Mucomyst, NAC) loading 140 mg/kg PO, then 70 mg/kg PO q4h x 17 doses (dilute to 5% sln)(follow acetaminophen levels) **OR** IV acetylcysteine 150 mg/kg in 200 ml NS or D5W IV over 15 min, followed by 50 mg/kg in 500 ml D5W, infused over 4h, followed by 100 mg/kg in 1000 ml of D5W over next 16h. Filter solution through 0.22 micron filter prior to administration. Complete all 17 doses, even after acetaminophen level falls below critical value.
   -Phytonadione 5 mg IV/IM/SQ (if PT >1.5 x control).
   -Fresh frozen plasma 2-4 U (if PT >3 x control).
   -Trimethobenzamide (Tigan) 100-200 mg IM/PR q6h prn nausea
10. **Extras:** ECG. Nephrology consult for possible hemodialysis or charcoal hemoperfusion. GI consult.
11. **Labs:** CBC, SMA 7&12, LFT's, LDH, amylase, PT/PTT, acetaminophen level now & in 4h (plot on nomogram; consider discontinuing treatment when below toxic). UA.
12. **Other Orders and Meds:**

THEOPHYLLINE OVERDOSE

1. **Admit to:** Medical intensive care unit.
2. **Diagnosis:** Theophylline overdose
3. **Condition:**
4. **Vital signs:** neurochecks; Call MD if:
5. **Activity:** bed rest
6. **Nursing:** ECG monitoring until level <20 mcg/ml, I&O, aspiration & seizure precautions. Insert 18 F Levin single lumes NG tube.
7. **Diet:** NPO
8. **IV Fluids:** D5½ NS at 125 cc/h
9. **Special Medications:**

-Activated Charcoal 50 gm PO q4-6h, followed by sorbitol cathartic (30 mls of 70% sln) regardless of time of ingestion, until theophylline level <20 mcg/ml. Maintain patient's head at 30-45 degrees to prevent aspiration of charcoal.

-Charcoal hemoperfusion (serum level >60 µg/ml, or signs of neurotoxicity, seizure, coma).

Seizure (support oxygenation & respirations): Phenobarbital or lorazepam, see page 77.

10. Extras: Portable CXR, ECG.

11. Labs: CBC, SMA 7, theophylline level now & in 4h; PT/PTT, liver panel. Monitor K, Mg, phosphorus, calcium. UA.

12. Other Orders and Meds:

TRICYCLIC ANTIDEPRESSANT OVERDOSE

1. Admit to: Medical Intensive Care unit.

2. Diagnosis: TCA Overdose

3. Condition:

4. Vital Signs: Neurochecks q1h.

5. Activity: Bedrest.

6. Nursing: ECG monitoring, QRS width measuring, I/O, pulse oximeter, aspiration and seizure precautions. Place 18 F Levin single lumen NG tube.

7. Diet: NPO

8. IV Fluids: NS at 100-150 cc/11.

9. Special Medications:
-Activated charcoal premixed with Sorbitol 50 Gms via NG tube q4-6h round-the-clock until TCA level decreases to therapeutic range.
Maintain patient's head at 30-45° angle to prevent charcoal aspiration.
-Magnesium citrate 300 mls NG x 1 dose.

10. Cardiac Toxicity: Alkalinization is a cardioprotective measure and it has no influence on drug elimination. Treatment goal is to achieve an arterial pH of 7.50-7.55.
-If mechanical ventilation is necessary hyperventilate to maintain desired pH.
-Administer sodium bicarbonate 50-100 mEq (1-2 amps or 1-2 mEq/Kg) IV over 5-10 min, followed by infusion of sodium bicarbonate 2 amps in D5W 1L at 100-150 cc/h. Adjust rate to maintain desired pH.

11. Seizures: Lorazepam or diazepam IV, followed by phenytoin (see page 77). Consider physostigmine 1-2 mg slow IV over 3-4 min if seizures continue.

12. Extras: CXR, ECG.

13. Labs: Urine toxicology screen, serum TCA levels if specific agent unknown, coagulation panel, hepatic panel, CBC, SMA-7, Mg, calcium, phos, UA.

14. Other Orders and Meds:

NEUROLOGY

ISCHEMIC STROKE
(Cerebral vascular accident)

1. **Admit to:**
2. **Diagnosis:** Ischemic stroke
3. **Condition:**
4. **Vital signs:** q1h with neurochecks q1h x 12h, then q6h; Call MD if BP >200/110, <90/60; P >120, <50; R>25, <10; T>38.5°C; or change in neuro status.
5. **Activity:** Bedrest for 24 hours, then up with assist & in chair tid if tolerated.
6. **Nursing:** HOB at 30 degrees, turn q2h when awake, range of motion exercises qid, Foley catheter, eggcrate mattress, sheepskin blanket, heal & elbow pads. Guaiac stools, I&O's.
7. **Diet:** NPO or dysphagia ground with thickened liquids.
8. **IV Fluids:** LR at 30 cc/h.
9. **Special Medications:**

Completed Ischemic Stroke:
   -Aspirin enteric coated 325 mg PO qd (non-hemorrhagic) **OR**
   -Ticlopidine (Ticlid) 250 mg PO bid.

Non-bacterial Cardiogenic, Progressing or Vertebrobasilar Ischemic Stroke:
   -Heparin, start immediately in non-hemorrhagic, small to moderate size infarcts) (controversial) 3000-5000 U IV (75 U/kg; reduce loading if ≥65 years) then 700-800 U/h (12 U/kg/h) IV (25,000 U in 500 ml D5W); adjust q6-12h until PTT 1.2-1.4 x control..
   -Warfarin 5.0-7.5 mg PO qd x 3d, then 2-4 mg (2-15 mg/d) PO qd. Maintain PT 1.2-1.3 x control (INR 2.0-2.5). Maintain warfarin for patients with evidence of cardiogenic or vertebrobasilar sources.

Increased intracranial pressure see page 76.

10. **Symptomatic Medications:**
   -Docusate sodium (Colace) 100-200 mg PO qhs.
   -Milk of magnesia 30 ml PO qd prn constipation **OR**
   -Bisacodyl (Dulcolax) 10-15 mg PO qhs or 10 mg PR prn **OR**
   -Casanthranol and docusate (Peri-Colace) 1 tab PO bid.
   -Ranitidine (Zantac) 50 mg IV q6-8h or 150 mg PO bid **OR**
   -Acetaminophen 325 mg 1-2 tabs PO/PR q4-6h prn temp > 100 or headache.
11. **Extras:** CXR, ECG, CT without contrast; MRI with or without gadolinium; carotid duplex; trans-esophageal echocardiogram, swallowing studies; 24 hour Holter monitor. Physical therapy, neurology, rehab med consults. Lumbar puncture after CT scan head, when clinical impression of subarachnoid hemorrhage but without CT scan confirmation.
12. **Labs:** CBC, SMA 7 & 12, lipid profile, blood C&S x 2, VDRL, FTA, osmolality, sickle prep, ESR, ANA, lupus anticoagulant, anticardiolipin; drug levels, PT/PTT, UA. Liver function tests.
13. **Other Orders and Meds:**

TRANSIENT ISCHEMIC ATTACK

1. **Admit to:**
2. **Diagnosis:** Transient ischemic attack
3. **Condition:**
4. **Vital signs:** q1h with neurochecks q1h x 12h, then q6h; Call MD if BP >160/90, <90/60; P >120, <50; R>25, <10; T>38.5°C; or change in neuro status.
5. **Activity:** Up in chair tid if tolerated.
6. **Nursing:** HOB at 30 degree. Guaiac stools.
7. **Diet:** Dysphagia ground with thickened liquids.
8. **IV Fluids:** Heplock with flush q shift.
9. **Special Medications:**

TRANSIENT ISCHEMIC ATTACK

-Aspirin 325 mg PO qd **OR**

-Ticlopidine (Ticlid) 250 mg PO bid **OR**

-Heparin (accelerating, recurrent TIA's; cardiogenic, or vertebrobasilar) 3000-5000 U IV (75 U/kg; reduce loading if ≥65 years) then 700-800 U/h (12 U/kg/h) IV infusion (25,000 U in 500 ml D5W); adjust q6-12h until PTT 1.2-1.3 x control.

-Warfarin (Coumadin) 5.0-7.5 mg PO qd x 3d, then 2-4 mg PO qd. Maintain PT 1.2-1.3 x control (INR of 2.0-2.5); maintain warfarin for patients with evidence of cardiogenic or vertebrobasilar sources.

10. **Symptomatic Medications:**

-Docusate sodium (Colace) 100-200 mg PO qhs.

-Milk of magnesia 30 ml PO qd prn constipation

-Ranitidine (Zantac) 50 mg IV q6-8h or 150 mg PO bid.

11. **Extras:** CXR, ECG, CT without contrast; carotid duplex, transcranial doppler, echocardiogram, 24h Holter. Physical therapy, neurology consults.
12. **Labs:** CBC, SMA 7 & 12, lipid profile, blood C&S x 2, VDRL, FTA, osmolality; drug levels, PT/PTT, UA. Liver function tests.
13. **Other Orders and Meds:**

SUBARACHNOID HEMORRHAGE

Treatment:

- HOB at 20 degrees, turn q2h when awake, range of motion exercises qid, Foley catheter, eggcrate mattress, sheepskin blanket, heal & elbow pads. Guaiac stools, I&O's.

-Keep room dark and quiet; no rectal exam; strict bedrest.

-Nimodipine (Nimotop) 60 mg PO or via NG tube q4h x 21d, must start within 96 hours.

-Propranolol 1-3 mg IV q6h or 10-60 mg PO qid, titrate to BP <160/90, hold

if hypotensive or bradycardic **OR**
-Nitroprusside sodium, 0.1-0.5 µg/kg/min (50-200 mg/250 ml NS), titrate.
-Phenobarbital 30-60 mg IV q12h prn mild sedation.
-Phenytoin (if seizure) IV load 15 mg/kg IV in NS (infuse at max 50 mg/min) in <u>dextrose free</u> IV, then 300 mg PO/IV qAM (4-6 mg/kg/d).
-Codeine 30-60 mg PO, IM, IV, or SQ q4-6h prn head pain.

11. Extras: CXR, ECG, CT without contrast; MRI angiogram; transcranial doppler, cerebral angiogram. Physical therapy, neurology, neurosurgery, rehab med consults. Lumbar puncture when CT scan without contrast is negative, and clinical impression of subarachnoid hemorrhage exists; check CSF cell count and xanthochromia.

12. Labs: CBC, SMA 7 & 12, lipid profile, blood C&S x 2, VDRL, FTA, osmolality; drug levels, UA. Liver function tests.

Other orders and meds:

INCREASED INTRACRANIAL PRESSURE

<u>Short-Term Measures to Reduce Pressure:</u>

-Restrict fluid to ½ maintenance, isotonic fluids. Head of bed at 30 degrees, head midline.
-Dexamethasone (Decadron) 10 mg IV or IM , followed by 4-6 mg IV, IM or PO q6h.
-Hyperventilation - maintain PCO_2 25-30 mm Hg.
-Mannitol, 100 gm (1-1.5 gm/kg) IV over 10-20 min (100 gm in 500 cc D5W), repeated q4-6h as needed; in less severe situations give 37.5-50 gm IV (0.5-1 gm/kg); keep osmolarity <315; do not give for >48h, used if dexa-methasone & hyperventilation unsuccessful with intracranial pressure monitor; rebound ↑ pressure may occur if discontinued.
-Furosemide (Lasix) 40-80 mg IV or PO qd-bid.
-Glycerol 1 gm/kg IV q6h.
-Pentobarbital (barbiturate coma) 7.5 mg/kg/h IV for 3h, then 2-3 mg/kg/h IV infusion, maintain pentobarbital level of 25-40 mg/L; requires intubation.
-Stat neurosurgery consult; possible placement ventricular device drainage with monitoring of intracranial pressure; possible evacuation of hematoma. The above measures have only a short term effect on ICP; primary etiology must be treated.

Other orders and meds:

SEIZURE & STATUS EPILEPTICUS

1. **Admit to:**
2. **Diagnosis:** Seizure
3. **Condition:**
4. **Vital signs:** q1h with neurochecks; Call MD if BP >160/90, <90/60; P >120, <50; R>25, <10; T>38.5°C; or any change in neurological status.
5. **Activity:** Bed rest
6. **Nursing:** Finger stick glucose now & qid. Seizure precautions, ECG & EEG monitoring.
7. **Diet:** NPO x 24h, then regular diet if alert.
8. **IV Fluids:** D5½NS at 100 cc/hr; change to hep-lock when taking PO.
9. **Special Medications:**

STATUS EPILEPTICUS (tonic-clonic)

1. Maintain airway, 100% O2 by mask, obtain brief history & physical, fingerstick glucose.
2. Secure IV access & draw labs (see below). If indicated, give **glucose, 50 ml of 50%** (1 amp) IV (in alcoholics give **thiamine (vitamin B1)**, 50 mg IV).
3. **Initial Control:**

   Lorazepam (Ativan) 4-8 mg IV at 1-2 mg/min. May repeat 4-8 mg q5-10min (max 80 mg/24h) **OR**

   Diazepam, 5-10 mg IV at 1-2 mg/min. Repeat 5-10 mg q5-10 min prn (max 100 mg/24h) **OR**

   Rectal Diazepam 30-80 mg (0.5-1 mg/kg; 6-16 ml of 5 mg/ml IV sln) PR with a small syringe 4-5 cm within rectum.

4. **Definitive Seizure Control: Consider Intubation:**
   1. **Phenytoin** 15-20 mg/kg load, in NS at 50 mg/min. Repeat 100-150 mg IV q30min, max 1.5 gms; monitor BP & ECG (QT interval). Hypotension may occur but should not preclude phenytoin; reduce the rate.
   2. **Phenobarbital** 120-260 mg (10-20 mg/kg) IV at 25-50 mg/min, repeat 20 mg/kg q15min; additional phenobarbital may be given, up to max of 30-60 mg/kg, then 60-130 mg IV q12h.

   If seizures persist, consider:
   3. **Induction of Coma: Pentobarbital** 10-15 mg/kg IV over 1-2h, then 1-1.5 mg/kg/h continuous infusion.
   4. Consider **General Anesthesia**; call anesthesiologist.

Primary Generalized Tonic-Clonic (Grand Mal)(low initial dose & titrate slowly):

-Carbamazepine (Tegretol) 200-400 mg PO tid **OR**
-Phenytoin PO/IV loading dose of 400 mg followed by 300 mg q4h x 2 doses (total of 1 g) then 300 mg qd or 100 mg tid or 200 mg bid.
-Felbamate (Felbatol) 1200-2400 mg PO qd in 3-4 divided doses; max 3600 mg/d. Adjunct therapy.

Partial Seizure, including Secondary Generalized

-Carbamazepine (Tegretol) 200-400 mg PO tid **OR**
-Phenytoin 300 mg PO/IV qd or 200 mg PO/IV bid **OR**
-Valproic acid (Depakene) 250-500 mg PO tid-qid [250 mg] or Divalproex

(Depakote) 15-30 mg/kg/d PO [125, 250, 500 mg]; less GI irritation than valproic acid **OR**

-Phenobarbital 30-120 mg PO/IV bid **OR**

-Primidone (Mysoline) 250-500 mg PO tid **OR**

-Felbamate (Felbatol) 1200-2400 mg PO qd in 3-4 divided doses; max 3600 mg/d. Adjunct therapy.

Absence (Petit Mal)

-Diazepam (status absence) 10-15 mg IV over 5 min **OR**

-Valproate, in status absence give 1000-3000 mg, diluted 1:1 in tap water as retention enema **OR** see oral dosage above.

Atypical Absence, Myoclonic, Atonic

-Valproate or divalproex, see above.

-Clonazepam (Klonopin)0.5-5 mg PO bid-qid.

10. Extras: MRI with & without gadolinium or C without contrast; EEG (awake & sleep); portable CXR, ECG, lumbar puncture (see page 74, 75, 76).

11. Labs: Stat CBC, SMA 7, glucose, Mg, calcium, phosphate, prolactin, CPK isoenzymes, liver panel, thyroid panel; blood alcohol; ammonia levels, VDRL, ABG, anticonvulsant levels. UA, urine culture, drug screen.

12. Other Orders and Meds:

ENDOCRINOLOGY

DIABETIC KETOACIDOSIS

1. **Admit to:**
2. **Diagnosis:** Diabetic ketoacidosis
3. **Condition:**
4. **Vital signs:** q1h, postural BP & pulse, neurochecks q4h. Call MD if BP >160/90, <90/60; P >140, <50; R>30, <10; T>38.5°C; or urine output < 20 cc/hr.
5. **Activity:** Bed rest with bedside commode.
6. **Nursing:** Daily weights, I&O. Foley to closed drainage. Record labs on flow sheet.
7. **Diet:** NPO.
8. **IV Fluids:**

0.5-5 L NS over 1-5h (≥16 gauge), infuse at 400-1000 mL/h until hemodynamically stable, then change to 0.45% saline at 150-400 cc/hr; keep urine output > 30-60 mL/h.

Add KCl when no ECG signs of hyperkalemia (peaked T) & urine output adequate, serum K+ ≤ 5.8 mEq/L.

      Concentration.......20-40 mEq KCl/L

      Rate.....................10-40 mEq KCl/hr

May use K phosphate, 20-40 mEq/L, in place of KCL if low phosphate.

Change to **D5** 0.45% saline with 20-40 mEq KCl or K phosphate/L when blood glucose 300-300.

9. **Special Medications:**
   - Oxygen at 2-5 L/min by NC or mask.
   - Insulin Regular (Humulin) 10-20 units (0.2 U/kg) IV bolus, then 5-10 U/h IV infusion (0.1 U/kg/h) (50 U in 250 ml of 0.9% saline at 25-75 ml/hr) (flush IV tubing with 20 ml of insulin sln before starting infusion). Adjust insulin infusion to decrease serum glucose by 100 mg/dl or less per hour.
   - Decrease Insulin to 2-4 U/hr, and change IV fluids to D5 0.45% saline with KCl or K phosphate 20-40 meq/l at 100-150 mls/hr, when serum glucose <250 mg/dl. Change to SC sliding scale when ketones & anion gap cleared; discontinue insulin drip 1-2h after SC dose.
   - Use 10% glucose at 50-100 ml/h if ketones and anion gap still present, & serum glucose <100 mg/dl while on insulin infusion. Continue insulin drip (with supportive glucose) until ketones and anion gap cleared.
   - Sodium bicarbonate (if pH <7.1) 44 mEq (50 ml) IV push or in 1 L 0.45% saline, infuse over 1h in place of NS, may repeat in 2 hrs. Correct to pH 7.1 with bicarbonate infusion or intermittent IVP.
   - Ranitidine (Zantac) 50 mg IV q6-8h.
10. **Extras:** Portable CXR, ECG.
11. **Labs:** Fingerstick glucose q1h x 6h, then q3-6h. SMA 7 & ketones q4-6h until anion gap and ketones negative. SMA 12, amylase, lipase, Hba1c, phosphate, CBC, Mg, calcium, ABG, blood and sputum C&S x 2. Consider cardiac enzymes q8h x 4. UA, urine protein, urine C&S, serum pregnancy test.
12. **Other Orders and Meds:**

NONKETOTIC HYPEROSMOLAR SYNDROME

1. **Admit to:**
2. **Diagnosis:** Nonketotic hyperosmolar syndrome
3. **Condition:**
4. **Vital signs:** q1h, postural BP & pulse, neurochecks q4h. Call MD if BP >160/90, <90/60; P >140, <50; R>25, <10; T>38.5°C; or urine output < 20 cc/hr.
5. **Activity:** Bed rest with bedside commode.
6. **Nursing:** I&O. Foley to closed drainage. Record labs on flow sheet.
7. **Diet:** NPO.
8. **IV Fluids:**
1-6 L NS over 1-7h (≥ 16 gauge) until no longer hypovolemic, then give 0.45% saline at 200-500 cc/hr. Maintain urine output ≥ 50 ml/h.
Add KCL when no ECG signs of hyperkalemia (peaked T), urine output adequate & serum K+ ≤ 5.0 mEq/L.

        Concentration....20-40 mEq KCl/L

        Rate.................10-40 mEq KCl/hr

May use K phosphate, 20-40 mEq/L, in place of KCL if low phosphate.
Change to **D5** 0.45% saline with 20-40 mEq KCl or K phosphate/L when blood glucose < 250.
9. **Special Medications:**
   -Insulin Regular 3-5 U/h IV infusion (50 U in 250 ml of 0.9% saline at 15-25 ml/hr) (flush IV tubing with 20 ml of sln before starting infusion).
   -Ranitidine (Zantac) 50 mg IV q6-8h.
10. **Extras:** portable CXR, ECG.
11. **Labs:** Fingerstick glucose q1h x 6, then q3-6h. SMA 7, osmolality. SMA 12, amylase, lipase, calcium, phosphate, ketones, HbA1C, CBC, blood and sputum C&S x 2. Cardiac enzymes. UA, urine C&S. Thyroid panel.
12. **Other Orders and Meds:**

THYROTOXICOSIS & HYPERTHYROIDISM

1. **Admit to:**
2. **Diagnosis:** Thyrotoxicosis
3. **Condition:**
4. **Vital signs:** q1h; Call MD if BP syst >160/90, <90/60; P >130, <50; R>25, <10; T>38.5°C
5. **Activity:** Bed rest
6. **Nursing:** Cooling blanket prn temp >39°C, triple blankets prn temp <36°C, I&O, seizure & aspiration precautions.
7. **Diet:** No added salt.
8. **IV Fluids:** Hep-lock

9. Special Medications:

Thyrotoxicosis & Hyperthyroidism:

- Propylthiouracil 300-400 mg PO, then 50-250 mg PO q4-8h, up to 1200 mg/d, usual maintenance dose 50 mg PO tid **OR**
- Methimazole (Thiamazole) 30-60 mg PO, then maintenance of 15 mg PO qd-bid **AND**
- Sodium iodine 1 gm IV q8h, 1h after propylthiouracil **OR**
- Potassium iodine (SSKI) 5-10 drops PO q8h, 1h after propylthiouracil **AND**
- Propranolol 10-40 mg PO q6h or 0.5-1 mg/min, max 2-10 mg IV q3-4h.
- Dexamethasone 1-2 mg IV or PO q6h.
- Acetaminophen 325 mg 1-2 tabs PO q4-6h prn temp >38°C.
- Triazolam (Halcion) 0.125-0.5 mg PO qhs prn sleep **OR**
- Lorazepam (Ativan) 1-2 mg IV/IM/PO q4-8h prn anxiety.

11. Extras: CXR PA & LAT, ECG, thyroid scan/radioactive iodine uptake, endocrine consult. If visual symptoms, obtain ophthalmology consult (rule out exophthalmos and/or optic neuropathy). (Possible radio-iodine vs subtotal thyroidectomy).

12. Labs: CBC, SMA 7&12, blood culture x 2, total T4, total T3, T3 resin uptake, TSH. Free T4 & T3, reverse T3, T4 binding globulin, T4 binding prealbumin, thyroid stimulating antibody, antithyroid microsomal, antithyroglobulin, cortisol, cardiac enzymes. UA. Beta HCG.

13. Other Orders and Meds:

MYXEDEMA COMA & HYPOTHYROIDISM

1. Admit to:

2. Diagnosis: Myxedema Coma

3. Condition:

4. Vital signs: q1h; Call MD if BP syst >160/90, <90/60; P >130, <50; R>25, <10; T>38.5°C

5. Activity: Bed rest

6. Nursing: Triple blankets prn temp <36°C, I&O, seizure & aspiration precautions.

7. Diet: NPO

8. IV Fluids: Hep-lock

9. Special Medications:

Myxedema Coma & Hypothyroidism:

- Volume replacement with NS at 200-300 cc/h & vasopressors if hypotensive. Correct hypoglycemia with 50% dextrose.
- Levothyroxine (Synthroid, T4, L-Thyroxine) 200-500 mcg IV over 2-4min, then 100-200 mcg PO or IV qd.
- Hydrocortisone 100 mg IV loading dose, then 50-100 mg IV q8h.

Hypothyroidism in Medically Stable Patient:

- Levothyroxine (Synthroid, T4) 25-50 mcg PO qd, increase by 25-50 mcg PO qd at 2-4 week intervals, to 50-200 mcg qd or 1.7 mcg/Kg/day, until T4/TSH normalized.

Hypothyroidism in Patient with Known Cardiac Disease:
- Levothyroxine (Synthroid, T4) 12.5 mcg PO qd; increase by 12.5-25 mcg qd at 3-4 week interval until full replacement reached (normalization of T_4/TSH); frequent cardiac follow up.

Hypothyroidism in Patient with Severe Medical or Surgical Stress (To Prevent Myxedema Coma):
- Levothyroxine 200-500 mcg IV over 2-4 min, followed by 100-200 mcg IV qd
  AND
- Hydrocortisone 100 mg IV q8h.

11. Extras: ECG, endocrine consult.

12. Labs: CBC, SMA 7&12, blood culture x 2, total T4, total T3, T3 resin uptake, TSH. Free T4 & T3, reverse T3, T4 binding globulin, T4 binding prealbumin, ABG, cortisol, cardiac enzymes, cholesterol. UA.

13. Other Orders and Meds:

NEPHROLOGY

RENAL FAILURE

1. **Admit to:**
2. **Diagnosis:** Renal Failure
3. **Condition:**
4. **Vital signs:** tid, postural vitals qAM, neurochecks, pulsus paradoxus; Call MD if V tach, or QRS complex > 0.14 sec; urine output < 20 cc/hr; BP >160/90, <90/60; P >120, <50; R>25, <10; T>38.5°C
5. **Allergies:** Avoid magnesium containing antacids, salt substitutes, NSAIDS, & other nephrotoxins. Avoid phosphates or potassium unless depleted.
6. **Activity:** Bed rest with bedside commode
7. **Nursing:** Daily weights, I&O, chart urine output q2h; if no urine output for 4h, I&O cath or Foley; Guiaic stools.
8. **Diet:** Maximum 2 gm sodium, potassium 2 g/day, & 20-80 gm protein (0.5-0.7 gm/kg/d) of 70% essential amino acids; 2,500 Cal/d (35-50 kcal/kg/d); 100 gm carbohydrate/d; phosphorus 800 mg/day maximum.
9. **IV Fluids:** D5W at TKO.
10. **Special Medications:**
    - Consider fluid challenge (to rule out pre-renal azotemia if not fluid overloaded) with 500-1000 ml NS IV over 30-60 min. In acute renal failure, I&O cath & check postvoid residual to rule out obstruction. Adjust all meds to creatinine clearance, & remove potassium from IV.
    - Consider administering diuretics after adequate central volume has been attained.
    - Furosemide (Lasix) 40-80 mg IV bolus over 10-60 min, double the dose if no response in 1-2h to total max 1000 mg/24h **May ADD**
    - Bumetanide (Bumex) 1-2 mg IV bolus over 1-20 min; double the dose if no response in 1-2 h to total max 10 mg/day.
    - Metolazone (Zaroxolyn) 5-10 mg PO (max 20 mg/24h) **OR**
    - Ethacrynic acid (Edecrin) 50-100 mg IV over 30 min **OR**
    - Mannitol 12.5-25 g (300-400 mg/kg) IV bolus (20-25% sln).
    - Calcium Acetate (PhosLo) 1-2 tabs PO with each meal (667 mg/tab, 169 mg elemental calcium q4h). Titrate dose to maintain serum phosphate <6.0 mg/dl.
    - Calcium carbonate (Oscal)(250 mg elemental Ca/625 mg tab or 500 mg Ca/1250 mg tab) 1-3 gm elemental calcium PO ac tid or Tums, 2 tabs PO bid. Keep calcium-phosphate product <70.
    - Hyperkalemia (see page 86).
    - Allopurinol (severe hyperuricemia) 100 mg PO qd.

Chronic Renal Failure:
    - Calcium acetate (PhosLo) 1-2 tabs PO with each meal (667 mg/tab, 169 mg elemental calcium q4h). Titrate dose to maintain serum phosphate <6.0 mg/dl.
    - Sodium bicarbonate 300-600 mg PO tid **OR**
    - Shohl's solution 15-30 ml diluted in water pc & hs (2 mEq bicarbonate/ml).
    - Erythropoietin (Epogen) 150 U/kg IV or SQ, 3 doses/week; reduce to 75

U/kg when Hct = 35, & titrate to Hct 32-38.

-Multivitamin (Nephro-Vite) PO qd.

-Folic acid 1 mg PO qd.

-Discontinue potentially nephrotoxic meds; aminoglycosides, NSAIDS, sulfonamides, IV contrast agents, cisplatin, cyclosporine, amphotericin.

11. Extras: CXR, KUB, ECG, renal ultrasound, Hippurate or technetium renal scan (may give Captopril 25 mg PO 1h prior to scan; contraindicated if bilateral renal artery stenosis), PPD, renal & dietetics consults.

12. Labs: CBC, reticulocytes, ABG, SMA 7 & 12, Mg, phosphate, calcium, uric acid, albumin, lipid panel. ESR, PT/PTT. ANA, rheumatoid, antiglomerular basement membrane, complement CH50, VDRL, ASO, streptizyme, HBsAg, serum protein electrophoresis, erythropoietin. UA with micro, urine Gram stain, C&S; 1st AM spot urine electrolytes, creatinine, pH, phosphate, osmolality, urine spot qualitative & quantitative protein, sulfosalicylic acid test (Bence Jones), Wright's stain, eosinophiles, electrophoresis. 24h urine protein, Cr, Na. Urine myoglobin (rule out rhabdomyolysis).

14. Other Orders and Meds:

NEPHROLITHIASIS

1. Admit to:

2. Diagnosis: Nephrolithiasis

3. Condition:

4. Vital signs: q4h x 12h, then q shift; Call MD if urine output < 30 cc/hr; BP >160/90, <90/60; T>38.5°C

5. Activity: Bed rest with bedside commode.

6. Nursing: Strain urine, I&O, urine output q4h, daily weights. Place Foley, if no urine for 4h. Urine hydrometer tid, instruct patient in usage (keep specific gravity >1.010).

7. Diet: Regular, 2-3 L fluids/d (maintain urine output of 2000 ml/d). Calcium restrict 400-600 mg/day (if absorptive hypercalciuria). Oxalate restrict 2 g/d (hyperoxaluria).

8. IV Fluids: IV D5½NS with 20 mEq KCL/L at 50-100 cc/hr.

9. Special Medications:

-Cefazolin (Ancef) 1-2 gm IV q8h

10. Symptomatic Medications:

-Meperidine (Demerol) 50-100 mg & hydroxyzine 25 mg IM q2-3h prn pain **OR**

-Morphine 4-8 mg slow IV push q5-15min prn pain **OR**

-Oxycodone (Roxicodone) 5 mg PO q4-6h prn pain **OR**

-Hydromorphone HCL (Dilaudid) 2-4 mg PO q4-6h prn pain **OR**

-Acetaminophen with codeine (Tylenol 4) 1-2 tabs PO q3-4h prn pain.

Note: If stone <5 mm without sepsis then discharge home with analgesics and increase PO fluids; if stone >10 mm (will not spontaneously pass) and/or fever increase WBC, then consider admission of patient with urology consult.

11. Extras: KUB, CXR, IVP, renal ultrasound, ECG.

12. Labs: CBC, SMA 6 & 12, calcium, uric acid, phosphorous, 1,25-vit D, UA with micro, urine C&S, PT/PTT. Urine, cystine (nitroprusside test), send stones for X-ray crystallography. If increased calcium, then check PTH level, urine pH. Outpatient testing: 24h urine calcium, uric acid, oxalate, creatinine, phosphate, magnesium cystine, sodium, citrate.

13. Other Orders and Meds:

HYPERCALCEMIA / HYPOCALCEMIA

1. Admit to:

2. Diagnosis: Hypercalcemia / Hypocalcemia

3. Condition:

4. Vital signs: q1h, neurochecks q4h; Call MD if BP >160/90, <90/60; P >120, <50; R>25, <10; T>38.5°C; or tetany or any abnormal mental status.

5. Activity: Hypocalcemia - up ad lib. Hypercalcemia - ambulate as often as possible, in chair at other times.

6. Nursing: Seizure precautions, tid weights, I & O.

7. Diet: Hypocalcemia - no added salt diet.
Hypercalcemia - restrict calcium to 400 mg/d, push PO fluids, 4-8 gm salt/d.

8. Special Medications:

Symptomatic HYPOcalcemia:

-Calcium chloride, 10% (270 mg calcium/10 ml vial) give 5-10 ml slowly over 5-10 min or dilute in 50-100 ml of D5 & infuse over 20 min, repeat q1-2h if symptomatic or q6-12h if asymptomatic **OR** infuse 3-4 ml of 10% calcium chloride in 500 ml NS over 8h. Maintain total serum calcium at 7-8 mg/dL; correct hyperphosphatemia before hypocalcemia. **OR**

-Calcium gluconate, 20 ml of 10% solution IV (2 vials)(90 mg elemental calcium/10 ml vial) infused over 10-15min, repeat q1-2h if symptomatic or q6-12h if asymptomatic **OR** infuse 1 vial in 500 ml of NS IV over 8h

Chronic HYPOcalcemia:

-Calcium carbonate (Oscal), (250 mg elemental Cal/625 mg tab or 500 mg Cal/1250 mg tab), 1-2 gm elemental calcium PO tid initially, then decrease to 0.5-1 gm elemental calcium PO tid. Maintain total serum calcium at 8.5-9 mg/dL. **OR**

-Calcium citrate (Citracal)(200 mg elemental Cal/1 gm tab), 3-5 gm PO q8h (600-1000 mg elemental Cal q8h).

-Calcitriol [1,25 $(OH)_2D_3$] (Rocaltrol), 0.25 µg PO qd **OR**

-Dihydrotachysterol [DHT] , 0.2-0.4 mg PO qd **OR**

-Calcifediol [25$(OH)D_3$] (Calderol), 50-100 µg PO qd **OR**

-Vitamin D2 (Ergocalciferol) 50,000-200,000 U PO qd.

-Hydrochlorothiazide 25-100 mg PO qd.

-Docusate sodium (Colace) 250 mg PO bid prn constipation.

HYPERcalcemia:

-1-4 L of 0.9 % saline at 150-600 cc/h IV until no longer hypotensive **THEN**

-Saline diuresis 0.9% or 0.45% saline infused at 300-600 cc/h to replace urine loss **AND**

-Furosemide (Lasix) 20-40 mg IV q2-12h. Maintain urine output of 200-500 ml/h; monitor I & O q2h, weigh pt q4h, measure serum Na, K+, Mg q4h, measure & replace urine Mg & K+ losses (empiric replacement: magnesium 15 mg/h & 10-30 mEq K+/h).

-Hydrocortisone (bone metastases), 5 mg/kg IV q8h, then prednisone 40-100 mg PO qd.

-Salmon calcitonin 4 IU/kg SQ or IM q12-24h, max 8 IU/kg IM q6h. Skin test with 0.1 ml of sln (10 IU/ml) intradermally first.

-Neutral phosphate (Nutra-Phos), 2-3 capsules (250 mg phosphate/capsule) PO tid-qid **OR** Phospho-Soda, 5 ml (645 mg phosphorus) PO tid-qid **OR** Sodium biphosphate (Fleet) enema 118 ml PR bid. Maintain phosphate 4-5 mg/dl & calcium-phosphate product <70.

-Etidronate disodium (Didronel) 7.5 mg/kg/d in 200 ml of 0.9% saline IV over 2h qd x 3-7d.

-Mithramycin (Mithracin) 25 mcg/Kg per day x 3-4 days (in 1000 mls D5W or NS over 4-6h). Use in hypercalcemia associated with malignancy unresponsive to other measures.

-Discontinue medication associated with increased calcium: Thiazide diuretics, lithium carbonate.

9. Extras: CXR, ECG, mammogram, renal ultrasound.

10. Labs: Total & ionized calcium, SMA 7 & 12, protein, albumin, phosphate, Mg, amylase, CPK, alkaline phosphatase, ABG, PTH, 1,25(OH) vitamin D, thyroid panel, globulin electrophoresis, prostate specific antigen, urine pH, electrolytes & Bence Jones proteins. 24h urine calcium, potassium, phosphate, magnesium, hydroxyproline. Prostate specific antigen.

11. Other Orders and Meds:

HYPERKALEMIA

1. Admit to:

2. Diagnosis: Hyperkalemia

3. Condition:

4. Vital signs: Vitals, neurochecks, postural BP, urine output q4h; Call MD if V tach, or QRS complex > 0.14 sec.

5. Activity: Bed rest; up in chair as tolerated.

6. Nursing: I&O, daily weights.

7. Diet: Regular, no salt substitutes.

8. IV Fluids: IV (see below).

9. Special Medications:

HYPERkalemia

-Consider discontinuing NSAIDS, ACE inhibitors, beta-blockers, K-sparing diuretics.

-Calcium gluconate 10% sln 10-30 ml IV over 2-5 min; second dose may be given in 5 min. Omit if dig toxicity suspected.

-NaHCO3 44-132 mEq (1-3 amps of 7.5%) IV over 5 min (give after calcium in separate IV), repeat in 10-15 min. Followed by infusion of 2-3 amps in

D5W, titrated over 2-4 h.
-Insulin 10-20 U regular in 500 ml of D10W IV over 1 hr or 10 units IV push
  with 1 amp 50% glucose (25 gm) over 5 min, repeat as needed.
-Kayexalate 15-50 gm in 100 ml of 20% sorbitol solution PO now & in 3-4h;
  up to 4-5 doses/d.
-Kayexalate retention enema 25-50 gm in 200 ml of 20% sorbitol; retain for
  30-60 min. (may use cleansing enema before).
-Furosemide 40-80 mg IV qd **OR**
-Hydrochlorothiazide 25-50 mg IV qd.
  -Consider emergent dialysis if cardiac complications or renal failure.
10. Extras: ECG, dietetics, nephrology consults.
11. Labs: CBC, platelets, SMA7, Mg, Cal, LDH, CPK isoenzymes, SMA-12,
lactate, ABG, renin, aldosterone. UA with micro, specific gravity, Na, K. bicarb,
Cl, pH, myoglobin, 24h urine K, Na, Cr, cortisol. Repeat electrolytes q2-4h until
stable.
13. Other Orders and Meds:

HYPOKALEMIA

1. Admit to:

2. Diagnosis: Hypokalemia

3. Condition:

4. Vital signs: Vitals, neurochecks, postural BP, urine output q4h; Call MD if:

5. Activity: Bed rest; up in chair as tolerated.

6. Nursing: I&O, daily weights.

7. Diet: Regular

8. IV Fluids: IV (see below).

9. Special Medications:

HYPOkalemia

If Serum K >2.5 mEq/L & ECG Changes are Absent:
-KCl 20-30 mEq/h IV sterile saline or IVPB in saline, up to 80 mEq/L as
  continuous IV infusion; may combine with 30-40 mEq PO q4h in addition
  to IV; total dose max is generally 100-200 mEq/d (3 mEq/kg/d).

Potassium <2.5 mEq/L & ECG Abnormalities Present:
-KCl IV 30-40 mEq/h & up to 80 mEq/L (glucose-free sln); may combine with
  PO 30-40 mEq q4h. Max daily dose IV (3 mEq/kg/d); give half over 24h.
-K-riders = 10-40 mEq in 100 ml of NS IVPB over 30-60 min, with primary
  line running at 80-125 cc/h.
  -Check for hypomagnesemia.

Chronic Therapy:
-KCl elixir 1-3 tablespoon qd-tid PO after meals (20 mEq/Tbsp 10% sln).
-Micro-K 10 mEq tabs 2-3 tabs tid PO after meals (40-100 mEq/d).
-Spironolactone 25-100 mg PO daily. **OR**
-Amiloride 5-10 mg PO qd.
-Check for hypomagnesemia.

HYPOkalemia with metabolic acidosis:
-Potassium citrate (1 mEq/ml) 15-30 ml in juice qid PO after meals.
-Potassium gluconate 15 ml in juice qid PO after meals (20 mEq/15 ml).
-Volume therapy with chloride containing sln; add bicarbonate if pH <7.2, 7.2
   Begin potassium Tx before starting bicarb Tx in separate IV line.
10. Extras: ECG, dietetics, nephrology consults.
11. Labs: CBC, SMA7, Mg, SMA 12, ABG, renin, aldosterone. UA with micro, osmolality, spec gravity, Na, K. bicarb, Cl, pH, 24h urine K, Na, Cr, protein, cortisol. Stool & urine sodium hydroxide test for phenolphthalein. Repeat electrolytes q2-4h until stable, beta hydroxysteroid dehydrogenase.
13. Other Orders and Meds:

HYPERMAGNESEMIA / HYPOMAGNESEMIA

1. **Admit to:**
2. **Diagnosis:** Hypermagnesemia / Hypomagnesemia
3. **Condition:**
4. **Vital signs:** q6h; Call MD if QRS >0.14 sec.
5. **Activity:** Up ad lib
6. **Nursing:** I & O, daily weights, seizure precautions. Hold all magnesium containing medications, including antacids.
7. **Diet:** regular
8. **IV Fluids:** see below
9. **Special Medications:**

HYPOmagnesemia:
   -Magnesium sulfate (severe hypomagnesemia <1.0) 1-2 gm (2-4 ml of 50% sln (8-16 mEq)) IV over 15 min, **OR**
   -Magnesium sulfate 1-6 gm in 500 ml D5W at 100 ml/h x 5h. Hold dose if no patellar reflex. (Estimation of Mg deficit = 0.2 x kg weight x desired increase in Mg concentration; give deficit over 2-3d) **OR**
   -Magnesium sulfate 1 gm (2 ml of 50% sln) IM q4-6h **OR**
   -Magnesium chloride (Slow-Mag) 65-130 mg (1-2 tabs) PO tid-qid (64 mg or 5.3 mEq/tab) **OR**
   -Magnesium oxide 1-2 tabs PO qd-qid (20.6 mEq Mg/416 mg tab) **OR**
   -Milk of magnesia 5 ml PO qd-qid.
   -Hold digoxin until hypomagnesemia resolved; monitor Ca+, K+.
   -**Medications Associated with Hypomagnesemia:** Loop diuretics, amino glycosides, amphotericin, cisplatin.

HYPERmagnesemia:
   -Saline diuresis 0.9% or 0.45% saline infused at 300-600 cc/h to replace urine loss **AND**
   -Calcium gluconate (10% sln; 1 gm (4.6 mEq) per 10 ml amp) 1-3 ampules added to saline infusate **AND**
   -Furosemide 20-40 mg IV q2h. Monitor I&O q2h, weigh pt q4h, serum Ca, Na, K, Mg q3h.
   -Magnesium of >9.0 requires stat hemodialysis (risk for cardiac arrest).

10. Extras: ECG
11. Labs: Magnesium, Calcium, SMA 7 & 12, thyroid panel, amylase, cortisol. Urine Mg, electrolytes, pH, 24h urine Mg, creatinine, calcium, potassium. PTH.
12. Other Orders and Meds:

HYPERNATREMIA

1. Admit to:
2. Diagnosis: Hypernatremia
3. Condition:
4. Vital signs: q4h, temp, neurochecks, postural vitals q4h; Call MD if BP >160/90, <70/50; P >140, <50; R>25, <10; T>38.5°C; seizure or any change in neurologic status.
5. Activity: Bed rest; up in chair as tolerated.
6. Nursing: Seizure precautions, I&O, weigh now & tid.
7. Diet: Fluids & Na (see below)
8. IV Fluids: IV (see below).
9. Special Medications:
Formulas: Serum osmolality = 2 [Na + K] + BUN/2.8 + glucose/18
HYPERnatremia:
  If volume depleted, give 0.5-3 L NS IV at 500 ml/hr until not orthostatic, then give D5W (if hyperosmolar) or D5½NS (if not hyperosmolar) IV or PO to replace half of body water deficit over first 24h (attempt to correct sodium at 1 mEq/L/h), then remaining deficit over next 1-2 days.
  Body water deficit (L) = $\dfrac{0.6(\text{weight kg})([\text{Na serum}]-140)}{140}$

HYPERnatremia with ECF volume excess:
  -Salt poor albumin (25%) 50-100 mls bid-tid x 48-72 h, if low oncotic pressure.
  -Furosemide 40-80 mg IV or PO qd-bid.
  -D5W to correct body water deficit (see above).
HYPERnatremia with Diabetes Insipidus:
  -D5W to correct body water deficit (see above).
  -Pitressin 5-10 U IM/IV q3-4h, keep urine specific gravity $\geq$1.010 **OR**
  -Desmopressin (DDAVP) 1-3 drops intranasal bid (10-20 µg/d), keep urine SG >1.010 **OR**
  -Chlorpropamide (central DI) 250-700 mg/d.
  -Hydrochlorothiazide (nephrogenic DI) 25-200 mg PO qd.
10. Extras: CXR, ECG.
11. Labs: SMA 7 & 12, osmolality, liver panel, ADH, thyroid panel, cortisol, renin, aldosterone. UA with micro, urine specific gravity. Urine osmolality, Na, K, bicarb, Cl, pH; 24h urine Na, K, Cr, protein, cortisol.
12. Other Orders and Meds:

HYPONATREMIA

1. **Admit to:**
2. **Diagnosis:** Hyponatremia
3. **Condition:**
4. **Vital signs:** q4h, temp, neurochecks, postural vitals q4h; Call MD if BP >160/90, <70/50; P >140, <50; R>25, <10; T>38.5°C; seizure or any change in neurologic status.
5. **Activity:** Bed rest; up in chair as tolerated.
6. **Nursing:** Seizure precautions, I&O, daily weights.
7. **Diet:** Fluids & Na (see below)
8. **IV Fluids:** IV (see below).
9. **Special Medications:**

For each 100 mg/dl ↑ in glucose, Na+ ↓ by 1.6 mEq/L.

HYPOnatremia with increased ECF & edema (Hypervolemia)(low osmolality <280, UNa <10 mmol/L: nephrosis, CHF, cirrhosis; UNa >20: acute/chronic renal failure):
  -Water restrict 0.5-1.5 L/d
  -2 gm salt/day diet.
  -Furosemide 40-80 mg IV or PO qd (20-600 mg/d).
  -If severe symptomatic hyponatremia, may require concurrent diuresis and sodium replacement.

HYPOnatremia with Isovolemia (low osmolality <280, UNa <10 mmol: water intoxication; UNa >20: SIADH, hypothyroidism, renal failure, Addison's disease, Stress, Drugs):
  -Furosemide 80 mg (1 mg/kg) IV qd-bid (20-600 mg/d) **AND**
  -0.9% saline with 20-40 mEq KCL/L at 65-150 cc/h (correct rate < 0.5 mEq/L/h).
  -Water restrict to 500-1500 ml/d.
  -8 gram/d salt diet (no salt restriction).
  -Demeclocycline (SIADH only) 150-300 mg PO q12h.

HYPOnatremia with Hypovolemia (low osmolality <280) UNa <10 mmol/L: vomiting, diarrhea, 3rd space/respiratory/skin loss; UNa >20 mmol/L: diuretics, renal injury, RTA, adrenal insufficiency, partial obstruction, salt wasting:
  If volume depleted, give 0.5-3 L of 0.9% saline at 500 cc/h until no longer orthostatic, then 0.9% saline (154 mEq/L) with 10-40 mEq KCl/L at 65-150 cc/h (determine volume as below) or 100 cc 3 % hypertonic saline over 5h.

Severe Symptomatic HYPOnatremia:
  If volume depleted, give 0.5-3 L of 0.9% saline at 500 cc/h until no longer orthostatic.
  Determine vol of 3% hypertonic saline (513 mEq/L) to be infused:

  Na (mEq) deficit = 0.6 x (wt kg)x(desired [Na] - actual [Na])

  $$\frac{\text{Volume of sln (L)}}{\text{Number of hrs}} = \frac{\text{Sodium to be infused (mEq)}}{\text{(mEq/L in sln) x Number of hrs}}$$

  Correct half of sodium deficit IV slowly over 24h to 120 mEq/L or increase by 12-20 mEq/L over 24h (1 mEq/L/h).

-Furosemide 40-80 mg IV or PO qd-bid.
-3% saline 100 cc over 4-6h repeat as needed (alternative method).
10. Extras: CXR, ECG, head/chest CT scan.
11. Labs: SMA 7 & 12, osmolality, triglyceride, cholesterol, albumin, liver panel, ADH, thyroid panel, cortisol, renin, aldosterone. UA with micro, urine specific gravity q4-6h. Urine osmolality, Na, K, bicarb, Cl, pH; 24h urine Na, K, Cr, protein, cortisol. Plasma osmolality.
12. Other Orders and Meds:

HYPERPHOSPHATEMIA / HYPOPHOSPHATEMIA

1. **Admit to:**
2. **Diagnosis:** Hyperphosphatemia / Hypophosphatemia
3. **Condition:**
4. **Vital signs:** qid
5. **Activity:** Up ad lib
6. **Nursing:** I&O, bid weights.
7. **Diet:** Hyperphosphatemia - restrict phosphorus to 0.7-1 gm/d. Hypophosphatemia - regular diet.
8. **IV Fluids:** see below.
9. **Special Medications:**

Mild HYPOphosphatemia:
-Na or K phosphate 0.25 mMoles/Kg IV infusion over 4 h (in 150-250 mls D5W or NS).
-Neutral phosphate (Nutra-Phos), 2 tab PO bid-tid (250 mg elemental phosphorus/tab, 7 mEq Na+ & 7 mEq K+/tab)**OR**
-Phospho-Soda (129 mg phosphorus & 4.8 mEq Na+/ml) 5 ml PO bid-tid.
-Milk 8 oz PO tid.
-Discontinue phosphate binding antacids.

Severe HYPOphosphatemia:
-Na or K phosphate 0.5 mMoles/Kg IV infusion over 4h (in 250 mls D5W or NS).
-Add potassium phosphate to IV solution in place of KCl (max 40 mEq/L infused at 100-150 ml/h) Max IV dose 7.5 mg phosphorus/kg/6-8h **OR** 2.5-5 mg elemental phosphorus/kg IV over 6-8h. Give as potassium or sodium phosphate (93 mg phosphate/ml & 4 mEq Na+ or K+/ml).
-Correct Ca+, Na+ or K+, I & 0 q2h, draw SMA 7, Mg, Cal, phosphate q3h. Do not mix calcium & phosphorus in same IV. Follow potassium level; if hyperkalemia, consider sodium phosphate supplementation.

Moderate HYPERphosphatemia:
-Aluminum hydroxide (Amphojel) 5-10 ml or 1-2 tablets PO ac tid **OR**
-Aluminum carbonate (Basaljel) 5-10 ml or 1-2 tablets PO ac tid **OR**
-Calcium carbonate (Oscal) (250 or 500 mg elemental calcium/tab) 1-2 gm elemental calcium PO ac tid. Keep calcium-phosphate product <70; start only if PO4 <5.5.
-Aluminum containing agents bind to unabsorbed phosphate in the GI

system, thus decreasing phosphate absorption. They have no direct effect on lowering elevated serum phosphate level. This is not an ion exchange.

Severe HYPERphosphatemia:
  -Volume expansion with 0.9% saline 1-3 L over 1-3h.
  -Acetazolamide (Diamox) 500 mg PO or IV q6h.
  -Consider dialysis.

10. Extras: CXR PA & LAT, ECG.

11. Labs: Phosphate, SMA 7 & 12, LDH, Mg, Cal, albumin, GGT, CPK, uric acid, ABG, 1,25(OH)vitamin D, PTH, urine electrolytes, pH. 24h urine phosphate, creatinine, potassium, UA with micro.

12. Other Orders and Meds:

RHEUMATOLOGY

SYSTEMIC LUPUS ERYTHEMATOSUS

1. **Admit to:**
2. **Diagnosis:** Systemic Lupus Erythematosus
3. **Condition:**
4. **Vital signs:** tid
5. **Allergies:** Avoid sulfonamides.
6. **Activity:**
7. **Nursing:** Guaiac all stools, dipstick urine.
8. **Diet:** No added salt, low psoralen diet.
9. **Special Medications:**
    -Aspirin 650-1300 mg PO qid (3.6-5.4 gm/d in divided doses) **OR**
    -Ibuprofen (Motrin) 300-600 mg PO tid-qid (max 2.4 g/d) **OR**
    -Indomethacin (Indocin) 25-50 mg tid-qid.
    -Hydroxychloroquine (Plaquenil) 200-600 mg/d PO
    -Prednisone 60-100 mg PO qd, may increase to 200-300 mg/d. Maintenance
        10-20 mg PO qd or 20-40 mg PO qOD **OR**
    -Methylprednisolone (pulse therapy) 500 mg IV over 30 min q12h for 3-5d,
        then prednisone 50 mg PO bid.
    -Cyclophosphamide (Cytoxan) 2 mg/kg/d PO or 0.5-1 gm/m^2 PO repeat
        monthly **OR**
    -Azathioprine (Imuran) 2 mg/kg/d PO.
    -Betamethasone dipropionate (Diprolene) 0.05% ointment **OR**
    -Triamcinolone acetonide (Aristocort)0.1% cream bid.
    -Vitamin D (steroid-induced osteopenia) 50,000 Units PO 2-3 times/week **OR**
    -Calcifediol 50 μg PO 3 times/week (max 350 μg/wk) **AND**
    -Calcium carbonate 1-1.5 gm PO qd.
    -Ranitidine (Zantac) 50 mg IV q6-8h or 150 mg PO bid
10. **Extras:** CXR PA, LAT & bilateral decubitus, ECG, intermediate strength
PPD with controls before starting steroids. Hippurate & technetium renal scan.
Nephrology, rheumatology consults.
11. **Labs:** CBC, platelets, SMA 7 & 12, blood C&S x 2. PT/PTT, bleeding time.
ESR, complement CH-50, C3, C4, C-reactive protein, C1q binding assay, LE
prep, Raji cells, cryoglobulins, haptoglobulin, Coomb's test, VDRL, rheumatoid
factor, ANA, anti-ds-DNA, anti-ss-DNA, SSB ab, anti-ribonucleoprotein, lupus
anticoagulant, anticardiolipin, anti-Sm, antihistone, anti-Ro, antinuclear
cytoplasmic, anti-smith; quantitative immunoglobulins; Lyme, HIV, rickettsii
titers. UA with micro, 24h urine protein, Cr.
12. **Other Orders and Meds:**

ACUTE GOUT ATTACK

1. **Admit to:**
2. **Diagnosis:** Acute gout attack
3. **Condition:**
4. **Vital signs:** q2h x 8h, then qid.
5. **Activity:** Bed rest with bedside commode
6. **Nursing:** Keep foot elevated, support sheets over foot, guaiac stools.
7. **Diet:** Low purine diet.
8. **Special Medications:**
   - Colchicine 2 tablets (0.5 mg or 0.6 mg) followed by 1 tablet q1h until relief, vomiting, diarrhea, or abdominal pain or max dose of 9.6 mg/24h. Then give maintenance colchicine 0.5-0.6 mg PO bid **OR**
   - IV Colchicine 2 mg diluted in 10-20 ml of NS & given slow IV push over 3-5 min (glucose free sln; observe IV for infiltration); saline & Hep-lock flush after each injection. Give additional 1-2 mg IV in 6h if needed. Max 4 mg/d (2 mg in renal, hepatic disease or elderly). Then give colchicine 0.5-0.6 mg PO bid.
   - Indomethacin (Indocin) 50 mg PO pc q6h x 2d, then 50 mg tid for 2 days, then 25 mg tid **OR**
   - Ketorolac (Toradol) 30-60 mg IM, then 15-30 mg IM q6h or 10 mg PO tid-qid. **OR**
   - Naproxen (Naprosyn) 500 mg tab PO tid for 2-3 days.
   - Methylprednisolone (SoluMedrol) 125 mg IV x 1 dose, **THEN**
   - Prednisone 40-60 mg PO qd x 5 days **OR**
   - Corticotropin 40 mcg IM with flair x 1.
   - Allopurinol 300 mg PO qd, may increase by 100-300 mg q2weeks **OR**
   - Probenecid 500 mg PO qd (do not use in acute phase), may increase by 500 mg every week to max of 3-4 gm/d.
   - Intra-articular injection with lidocaine/marcaine +/- corticosteroids (triamcinolone on hexacetonide (Aristospan)).
9. **Symptomatic Medications:**
   - Ranitidine (Zantac) 150 mg PO bid.
   - Acetaminophen/codeine (Tylenol 3) 1-2 tabs PO q4-6h prn pain.
10. **Labs:** CBC, SMA 7, uric acid, ESR. UA with micro. 24h urine for creatinine & uric acid. Synovial fluid for light and polarizing microscope analysis for crystals, C&S, Gram stain, glucose, protein, cell count, pH. X-ray views of joint.
11. **Other Orders and Meds:**

FORMULAS

A-a gradient = $[(P_B - PH_2O) FiO_2 - PCO_2/R] - PO_2$ arterial

$\qquad$ = $(713 \times FiO_2 - pCO_2/0.8) - pO_2$ arterial

P_B = 760 mmHg; PH_2O = 47 mmHg; R ≈ 0.8
normal Aa gradient <10-15 mmHg (room air)

Arterial oxygen capacity = (Hgb(gm)/100 ml) x 1.36 ml O2/gm Hgb

Arterial O2 content = 1.36(Hgb)(SaO2)+0.003(PaO2)= NL 20 vol%

O2 delivery = CO x arterial O2 content = NL 640-1000 ml O2/min

Cardiac output = HR x stroke volume

$$CO \text{ L/min} = \frac{125 \text{ ml O2/min/M}^2}{8.5\{(1.36)(Hgb)(SaO2) - (1.36)(Hgb)(SvO2)\}} \times 100$$

Note: 125 is a crude estimate for normals
Normal CO = 4-6 L/min

Na (mEq) deficit = 0.6 x (wt kg) x (desired [Na] - actual [Na])

$$SVR = \frac{MAP - CVP}{CO_{L/min}} \times 80 = NL \ 800\text{-}1200 \ dyne/sec/cm^2$$

$$PVR = \frac{PA - PCWP}{CO_{L/min}} \times 80 = NL \ 45\text{-}120 \ dyne/sec/cm^2$$

$$GFR \ ml/min = \frac{(140 - age) \ x \ wt \ in \ Kg}{72 \ (males) \ x \ serum \ Cr \ (mg/dl)}$$
$$85 \ (females) \ x \ serum \ Cr \ (mg/dl)$$

$$Creatinine \ clearance = \frac{U \ Cr \ (mg/100 \ mL) \ x \ U \ vol \ (mL)}{P \ Cr \ (mg/100 \ mL) \ x \ time \ (1440 \ min \ for \ 24h)}$$

Normal creatinine clearance = 100-125 ml/min(males), 85-105(females)

$$Body \ water \ deficit \ (L) = \frac{0.6(weight \ kg)([measured \ serum \ Na]-140)}{140}$$

$$Serum \ Osmolality = 2 \ [Na] + \frac{BUN}{2.8} + \frac{Glucose}{18} = 270\text{-}290$$

Na (mEq) deficit = 0.6 x (wt kg) x (desired [Na] - actual [Na])

$$Fractional \ excreted \ Na = \frac{U \ Na/ \ Serum \ Na}{U \ Cr/ \ Serum \ Cr} \times 100 = NL <1\%$$

Anion Gap = Na + K - (Cl + HCO3)

For each 100 mg/dl ↑ in glucose, Na+ ↓ by 1.6 mEq/L.

Corrected serum Ca+ (mg/dl) = measured Ca mg/dl + 0.8 x (4 - albumin g/dl)

Ideal body weight males = 50 kg for first 5 feet of height + 2.3 kg for each additional inch.

Ideal body weight females = 45.5 kg for first 5 feet + 2.3 kg for each additional inch.

Basal energy expenditure (BEE):
Males=66 + (13.7 x actual weight Kg) + (5 x height cm)-(6.8 x age)
Females= 655+(9.6 x actual weight Kg)+(1.7 x height cm)-(4.7 x age)

Nitrogen Balance = Gm protein intake/6.25 - urine urea nitrogen - (3-4 gm/d insensible loss)

Predicted Maximal Heart Rate = 220 - age

Normal ECG Intervals (sec)

PR	0.12-0.20
QRS	0.06-0.08
Heart rate/min	**Q-T**
60	0.33-0.43
70	0.31-0.41
80	0.29-0.38
90	0.28-0.36
100	0.27-0.35

DRUG LEVELS OF COMMON MEDICATIONS

DRUG	THERAPEUTIC RANGE*
Amikacin	Peak 25-30; trough <10 mcg/ml
Amitriptyline	100-250 ng/ml
Carbamazepine	4-10 mcg/ml
Chloramphenicol	Peak 10-15; trough <5 mcg/ml
Desipramine	150-300 ng/ml
Digitoxin	10-30 ng/ml
Digoxin	0.8-2.0 ng/ml
Disopyramide	2-5 mcg/ml
Doxepin	75-200 ng/ml
Ethosuximide	40-100 mcg/ml
Flecainide	0.2-1.0 mcg/ml
Gentamicin	Peak 6.0-8.0; trough <2.0 mcg/ml
Imipramine	150-300 ng/ml
Lidocaine	2-5 mcg/ml
Lithium	0.5-1.4 meq/L
Nortriptyline	50-150 ng/ml
Phenobarbital	10-30 meq/ml
Phenytoin**	8-20 mcg/ml
Procainamide	4.0-8.0 mcg/ml
Quinidine	2.5-5.0 mcg/ml
Salicylate	15-25 mg/dl
Streptomycin	Peak 10-20; trough <5 mcg/ml
Theophylline	8-20 mcg/ml
Tocainide	4-10 mcg/ml
Valproic acid	50-100 mcg/ml
Vancomycin	Peak 30-40; trough <10 mcg/ml

* The therapeutic range of some drugs may vary depending on the reference lab used.
** Therapeutic range of phenytoin is 4-10 mcg/ml in presence of significant azotemia and/or hypoalbuminemia.

COMMON ABBREVIATIONS

aa	of each		PO	orally
ac	before meals		PR	per rectum
ad	right ear		prn	as needed
ad lib	as needed or desired		q	every
am	morning		qAM	every morning
AMA	against medical advice		qd	every day
amt	amount		qh	every hour
ante	before		qhs	every night before bedtime
as, al	left ear		qid	4 times a day
au	both ears		qOD	every other day
aq	water		q 6 h	every 6 hours
bid	twice a day		qs	quantity sufficient
BP	blood pressure		sat	saturated
c	with		SL	place under tongue
cc	cubic centimeter		sob	shortness of breath
caps	capsules		sol	solution
cm	centimeter		SQ	under the skin
c/o	complaint of		ss	one-half
dil	dilute		stat	immediately
dr	dram		tab	tablet
Etoh	alcohol		tbsp	tablespoon
exp	expired		temp	temperature
F	Fahrenheit		tid	three times a day
Fe	iron		tr or tinc	tincture
fl	fluid		tsp	teaspoon
gm	gram		ung	ointment
gr	grain		USP	United States Pharmacopeia
gt	drop		Ut Dict	as directed
gtt	drops		vag	vaginal
H, h .hr	hour		Vol	volume
H20	water		x	times
hr	hour			
hs	bedtime, hour of sleep			
I M	intramuscular			
K	potassium			
liq	liquid			
Mg	magnesium			
mg, mgm	milligram			
MgSO4	Magnesium Sulfate			
mm	millimeter			
MOM	Milk of Magnesia			
NG	nasal tube			
NKA	no known allergies			
NPO	nothing per mouth			
OD	right eye			
oint	ointment			
OS, OL	left eye			
OU	each eye			
oz	ounce			
p	after			
PB	phenobarbital			
pc	after meals			
per	by			
pm	afternoon			

Never use an abbreviation for "units"

TABLE OF METRIC DOSES WITH APPROXIMATE APOTHECARY EQUIVALENTS

Liquid Measure

Metric		Approximate Apothecary Equivalents	
1000	ml.	1	quart
750	ml.	1 ½	pints
500	ml.	1	pint
250	ml.	8	fluid ounces
200	ml.	7	fluid ounces
100	ml.	3 ½	fluid ounces
50	ml.	1 ¾	fluid ounces
30	ml.	1	fluid ounce
15	ml.	4	fluid drams
10	ml.	2 ½	fluid drams
8	ml.	2	fluid drams
5	ml.	1 ¼	fluid drams
4	ml.	1	fluid dram
3	ml.	45	minims
2	ml.	30	minims
1	ml.	15	minims
0.6	ml.	10	minims
0.5	ml.	8	minims
0.3	ml.	5	minims
0.25	ml.	4	minims
0.2	ml.	3	minims
0.1	ml.	1½	minims
0.06	ml.	1	minim
0.05	ml.	¾	minim
0.03	ml.	½	minim

Weight

Metric		Approximate Apothecary Equivalents	
30	Grn	1	ounce
15	Gm	4	drams
10	Gm	2 ½	drams
7.5	Gm	2	drams
6	Gm	90	grains
5	Gm	75	grains
4	Gm	60	grains (1 dram)
3	Gm	45	grains
2	Gm	30	grains (½ dram)
1.5	Gm	22	gains
1	Gm	15	gains

REGISTRATION CARD AND ORDER FORM

Submission of this form (with or without ordering) entitles you to receive FREE drug updates, revision announcements, catalogs and discounts on our publications.

Current Clinical Strategies, Prescription Writer Computer Program
Prescription Writing System and Record Manager. Produces legible prescriptions in seconds, and keeps an updated list of each patient's medications. Includes a database of over 1500 dosages. Installs on any IBM PC, AT or above computer; dot matrix or laser printer. No special paper required, Rx paper included. Available 3/1/94.
Please circle one: 5¼   3½ inch diskettes   #___ x $55.00

Current Clinical Strategies,
   Physician's Drug Reference (available February 15, 1994)   #___ x $8.75

Handbook of Anesthesia
   Mark Ezekiel (available January 30, 1994)   #___ x $8.75

Manual of HIV/AIDS Therapy
   Laurence Peiperl   #___ x $8.75

Current Clinical Strategies,
   MEDICINE, Paul D. Chan,   NEW 1994 edition   #___ x $8.75

Current Clinical Strategies,
   GYNECOLOGY & OBSTETRICS, NEW 1994 edition   #___ x $10.75

Current Clinical Strategies,
   PEDIATRICS, NEW 1994 edition   #___ x $8.75

FAMILY MEDICINE, NEW 1994 edition
   Pediatrics, Medicine, Gynecology, Obstetrics   #___ x $26.25

DIAGNOSTIC HISTORY & PHYSICAL
   EXAMINATION in MEDICINE   #___ x $8.75

OUTPATIENT MEDICINE   #___ x $8.75

CRITICAL CARE MEDICINE.   #___ x $8.75

PSYCHIATRY   #___ x $8.75

Handbook of Psychiatric Drug Therapy   #___ x $8.75

Current Clinical Strategies,
   SURGERY   #___ x$8.75

Total ___

Prices are in US dollars & include shipping. Other countries, send equivalent amount in foreign check. Prices and availability subject to change without notice.
Order by Phone: 1-800-331-8227 (add $1.50 COD charge per order; a bill will be sent with order)
Order by Mail. Send order & check payable to:

Current Clinical Strategies Publishing
9550 Warner Ave, Suite 250
Fountain Valley, Ca USA 92708-2822

Return Address: _____

_____

_____

Phone Number: (_____) _____
Please complete reverse side.

Is this book sold at your local medical book store? ___ yes ___ no

Name, address and phone number of bookstore:

_____

_____

_____

Receive $8.75 off your order if this book is not available in your local bookstore. Receive discount by enclosing the business card or letterhead stationary of the bookstore manager with your order. Take $8.75 off total.
Readers are encouraged to write additional sections or to submit their own manuscripts for publication.

Comments:

We appreciate your comments -- good and bad -- about our books and software. We would also like to know what features you want added to future editions.

Current Clinical Strategies Publishing
9550 Warner Avenue, Suite 250, Fountain Valley, CA 92708-2822
Phone: 1-800-331-8227

Suggested additions, problems or criticisms: _____

Albuterol/Proventil nebs 2.5 ml
2 q 4°!
Theodur 300mg po bid

_____

_____

_____

_____

_____

_____

_____

_____

_____

REGISTRATION CARD AND ORDER FORM

Submission of this form (with or without ordering) entitles you to receive FREE drug updates, revision announcements, catalogs and discounts on our publications.

Current Clinical Strategies, Prescription Writer Computer Program
Prescription Writing System and Record Manager. Produces legible prescriptions in seconds, and keeps an updated list of each patient's medications. Includes a database of over 1500 dosages. Installs on any IBM PC, AT or above computer; dot matrix or laser printer. No special paper required, Rx paper included. Available 3/1/94.
Please circle one: 5¼   3½ inch diskettes   #___ x $55.00

Current Clinical Strategies,   #___ x $8.75
  Physician's Drug Reference (available February 15, 1994)

Handbook of Anesthesia   #___ x $8.75
  Mark Ezekiel (available January 30, 1994)

Manual of HIV/AIDS Therapy   #___ x $8.75
  Laurence Peiperl

Current Clinical Strategies,   #___ x $8.75
  MEDICINE, Paul D. Chan,   NEW 1994 edition

Current Clinical Strategies,   #___ x $10.75
  GYNECOLOGY & OBSTETRICS, NEW 1994 edition

Current Clinical Strategies,   #___ x $8.75
  PEDIATRICS, NEW 1994 edition

FAMILY MEDICINE, NEW 1994 edition   #___ x $26.25
  Pediatrics, Medicine, Gynecology, Obstetrics

DIAGNOSTIC HISTORY & PHYSICAL   #___ x $8.75
  EXAMINATION in MEDICINE

OUTPATIENT MEDICINE   #___ x $8.75

CRITICAL CARE MEDICINE.   #___ x $8.75

PSYCHIATRY   #___ x $8.75

Handbook of Psychiatric Drug Therapy   #___ x $8.75

Current Clinical Strategies,   #___ x $8.75
  SURGERY
                                                   Total ___

Prices are in US dollars & include shipping. Other countries, send equivalent amount in foreign check. Prices and availability subject to change without notice.
Order by Phone: 1-800-331-8227 (add $1.50 COD charge per order; a bill will be sent with order)
Order by Mail. Send order & check payable to:

   Current Clinical Strategies Publishing
   9550 Warner Ave, Suite 250
   Fountain Valley, Ca USA 92708-2822

Return Address: _____

                       _____

                       _____

Phone Number: (_____)_____
Please complete reverse side.

Is this book sold at your local medical book store? ___ yes ___ no

Name, address and phone number of bookstore:

_____

_____

_____

Receive $8.75 off your order if this book is not available in your local bookstore. Receive discount by enclosing the business card or letterhead stationary of the bookstore manager with your order. Take $8.75 off total.

Readers are encouraged to write additional sections or to submit their own manuscripts for publication.

Comments:

We appreciate your comments -- good and bad -- about our books and software. We would also like to know what features you want added to future editions.

Current Clinical Strategies Publishing
9550 Warner Avenue, Suite 250, Fountain Valley, CA 92708-2822
Phone: 1-800-331-8227

Suggested additions, problems or criticisms: _____

_____

_____

_____

_____

_____

_____

_____

_____

_____

_____

_____

_____

_____

REGISTRATION CARD AND ORDER FORM

Submission of this form (with or without ordering) entitles you to receive FREE drug updates, revision announcements, catalogs and discounts on our publications.

Current Clinical Strategies, Prescription Writer Computer Program
Prescription Writing System and Record Manager. Produces legible prescriptions in seconds, and keeps an updated list of each patient's medications. Includes a database of over 1500 dosages. Installs on any IBM PC, AT or above computer; dot matrix or laser printer. No special paper required, Rx paper included. Available 3/1/94.

Please circle one: 5¼   3½ inch diskettes   #___ x $55.00

Current Clinical Strategies,   #___ x $8.75
    Physician's Drug Reference (available February 15, 1994)

Handbook of Anesthesia   #___ x $8.75
    Mark Ezekiel (available January 30, 1994)

Manual of HIV/AIDS Therapy   #___ x $8.75
    Laurence Peiperl

Current Clinical Strategies,   #___ x $8.75
    MEDICINE, Paul D. Chan, NEW 1994 edition

Current Clinical Strategies,   #___ x $10.75
    GYNECOLOGY & OBSTETRICS, NEW 1994 edition

Current Clinical Strategies,   #___ x $8.75
    PEDIATRICS, NEW 1994 edition

FAMILY MEDICINE, NEW 1994 edition   #___ x $26.25
    Pediatrics, Medicine, Gynecology, Obstetrics

DIAGNOSTIC HISTORY & PHYSICAL   #___ x $8.75
    EXAMINATION in MEDICINE

OUTPATIENT MEDICINE   #___ x $8.75

CRITICAL CARE MEDICINE.   #___ x $8.75

PSYCHIATRY   #___ x $8.75

Handbook of Psychiatric Drug Therapy   #___ x $8.75

Current Clinical Strategies,   #___ x $8.75
    SURGERY

       Total ____

Prices are in US dollars & include shipping. Other countries, send equivalent amount in foreign check. Prices and availability subject to change without notice.

Order by Phone: 1-800-331-8227 (add $1.50 COD charge per order; a bill will be sent with order)

Order by Mail. Send order & check payable to:

    Current Clinical Strategies Publishing
    9550 Warner Ave, Suite 250
    Fountain Valley, Ca USA 92708-2822

Return Address: _____
                   _____
                   _____

Phone Number: (_____)_____
Please complete reverse side.

Is this book sold at your local medical book store? ___ yes ___ no

Name, address and phone number of bookstore:

_____

_____

Receive $8.75 off your order if this book is not available in your local bookstore. Receive discount by enclosing the business card or letterhead stationary of the bookstore manager with your order. Take $8.75 off total.

Readers are encouraged to write additional sections or to submit their own manuscripts for publication.

Comments:

We appreciate your comments -- good and bad -- about our books and software. We would also like to know what features you want added to future editions.

Current Clinical Strategies Publishing
9550 Warner Avenue, Suite 250, Fountain Valley, CA 92708-2822
Phone: 1-800-331-8227

Suggested additions, problems or criticisms: _____

_____

_____

_____

_____

_____

_____

_____

_____

_____

_____

REGISTRATION CARD AND ORDER FORM

Submission of this form (with or without ordering) entitles you to receive FREE drug updates, revision announcements, catalogs and discounts on our publications.

Current Clinical Strategies, Prescription Writer Computer Program
Prescription Writing System and Record Manager. Produces legible prescriptions in seconds, and keeps an updated list of each patient's medications. Includes a database of over 1500 dosages. Installs on any IBM PC, AT or above computer; dot matrix or laser printer. No special paper required. Rx paper included. Available 3/1/94.
Please circle one: 5¼   3½ inch diskettes   #___ x $55.00

Current Clinical Strategies,
Physician's Drug Reference (available February 15, 1994)   #___ x $8.75

Handbook of Anesthesia
Mark Ezekiel (available January 30, 1994)   #___ x $8.75

Manual of HIV/AIDS Therapy
Laurence Peiperl   #___ x $8.75

Current Clinical Strategies,
MEDICINE, Paul D. Chan,   NEW 1994 edition   #___ x $8.75

Current Clinical Strategies,
GYNECOLOGY & OBSTETRICS, NEW 1994 edition   #___ x $10.75

Current Clinical Strategies,
PEDIATRICS, NEW 1994 edition   #___ x $8.75

FAMILY MEDICINE, NEW 1994 edition
Pediatrics, Medicine, Gynecology, Obstetrics   #___ x $26.25

DIAGNOSTIC HISTORY & PHYSICAL
EXAMINATION in MEDICINE   #___ x $8.75

OUTPATIENT MEDICINE   #___ x $8.75

CRITICAL CARE MEDICINE.   #___ x $8.75

PSYCHIATRY   #___ x $8.75

Handbook of Psychiatric Drug Therapy   #___ x $8.75

Current Clinical Strategies,
SURGERY   #___ x$8.75

                                                       Total _____

Prices are in US dollars & include shipping. Other countries, send equivalent amount in foreign check. Prices and availability subject to change without notice.
Order by Phone: 1-800-331-8227 (add $1.50 COD charge per order; a bill will be sent with order)
Order by Mail. Send order & check payable to:

Current Clinical Strategies Publishing
9550 Warner Ave, Suite 250
Fountain Valley, Ca USA 92708-2822

Return Address: _____
                      _____
                      _____

Phone Number: (_____) _____
Please complete reverse side.

Is this book sold at your local medical book store? ___ yes ___ no

Name, address and phone number of bookstore:

_____

_____

_____

Receive $8.75 off your order if this book is not available in your local bookstore. Receive discount by enclosing the business card or letterhead stationary of the bookstore manager with your order. Take $8.75 off total.

Readers are encouraged to write additional sections or to submit their own manuscripts for publication.

Comments:

We appreciate your comments -- good and bad -- about our books and software. We would also like to know what features you want added to future editions.

Current Clinical Strategies Publishing
9550 Warner Avenue, Suite 250, Fountain Valley, CA 92708-2822
Phone: 1-800-331-8227

Suggested additions, problems or criticisms: _____

_____

_____

_____

_____

_____

_____

_____

_____

_____

_____